I0414289

# Paleo Diet for Beginners:

80 Healthy Paleo Recipes and 31 Proven Steps to Loose Weight

*By Rebecca Publishing*

# Paleo Diet for Beginners:

80 Healthy Paleo Recipes and 31 Proven Steps to Loose Weight

# Paleo Diet for Beginners:

80 Healthy Paleo Recipes and 31 Proven Steps to Loose Weight

**Disclaimer**

All the material contained in this book is provided for informational and educational purposes only. No responsibility can be taken for any outcomes resulting from the use of this material.

While every attempt has been made to provide information that is both accurate and effective, the author does not assume any responsibility for the accuracy or use/misuse of this information.

# Paleo Diet for Beginners:

80 Healthy Paleo Recipes and 31 Proven Steps to Loose Weight

**About the author**!

I am a newbie to publishing business, but I have a lot of information to tell you. I have been studying healthy way of eating from leading nutritionist in Europe and I have a lot of useful information on this topic. I have lost more than 20 kilos so I can provide you with a lot of practical tips on this matter.

My story is also very bright, after giving birth to a child; I have gained a lot of extra weight. It was simply impossible to look into the mirror, but I decided to do my best to return to my previous shape. I have tried swimming, jogging, different diets like Dukan, Sugar Free Diet, Kremlyovskaya Diet etc. These diets forced me to starving and nothing more.  I saw and fell the best result after following the Paleo Diet. This diet helped me to loose ALL my extra weight this is more than 20 kilos/44 pounds and I feel myself much healthier now! So, Let's start my explanation of what is it – paleo diet and the main aspects of it.

# Paleo Diet for Beginners:

## 80 Healthy Paleo Recipes and 31 Proven Steps to Loose Weight

Introduction

Thank you for downloading of my book - Paleo Diet for Beginners: 80 Healthy Paleo Recipes and 31 Proven Steps to Loose Weight. I have combined two of my books and make more convenient box set where you can find all healthy and affordable paleo recipes.

If you wish to loose weight and stay healthy, like people say, to kill two birds with one stone, then this book is the proper thing for you. So let`s begin our way to healthy life with beautiful body? There are a lot of useful information and a lot of mouth-watering recipes below.

# Paleo Diet for Beginners:

## 80 Healthy Paleo Recipes and 31 Proven Steps to Loose Weight

## The History of Paleo Diet

I would like to tell you some words about the history of the Paleo Diet. This diet was developed and presented in the 1970s by the doctor, actually gastroenterologist. The name of this person is Walter Voegtlin. The main suggestion of him was to eat like our forefathers and become healthier, stronger and lean in such a way. What is more he claimed that this diet can reduce a lot of health problems such as diabetes, obesity and even Crohn`s disease. . It helps you to better your mental health. This diet is also a great way to make your face look better without spots and acne. What is more paleo diet makes a positive affect to your immune system as well as your digestion system. To crown it all the paleo diet can help you to minimize your blood pressure and better your sleep.

Mr Walter Voegtlin claimed, the main principles of this diet is to eat everything what our Paleolithic men consumed. These are mainly the following products: meats and fish (because it was easy to hunt for) also nuts, seeds, different fruits and vegetable. Everything is simple.

Now I would like to proceed to the first chapter where I am going to list all 31 proven steps on paleo diet which will bring you to healthy way of living and beautiful shape.

# Paleo Diet for Beginners:

## 80 Healthy Paleo Recipes and 31 Proven Steps to Loose Weight

## Table of Contents

# Paleo Diet for Beginners:

## 80 Healthy Paleo Recipes and 31 Proven Steps to Loose Weight

# Paleo Diet for Beginners:

## 80 Healthy Paleo Recipes and 31 Proven Steps to Loose Weight

# Paleo Diet for Beginners:

## 80 Healthy Paleo Recipes and 31 Proven Steps to Loose Weight

# Paleo Diet for Beginners:

80 Healthy Paleo Recipes and 31 Proven Steps to Loose Weight

Chapter 1

*31 Proven Steps of Paleo Diet for Beginners*

1. You can replace sugar by the honey. This will add more vitamins into your daily menu and will not allow you to gain weight.

2. You can replace grains with all kinds of vegetables. You can eat them either fresh or frozen. Sweet potatoes and yams are allowed as well.

3. You can replace all sort of oils like corn oil or soy oil by home – made mayonnaise. Avoid eating fried food it affects destroying to your digestive organs.

4. Eat a lot of meat, it is better to eat meat from pastured animals. There are a lot of meat, which contains antibiotics; hormones try to avoid buying such sort of meat.

5. Try to include intake of eggs into your weekly rations, as eggs contain omega 3. You can enjoy different sorts of egg like: duck egg, chicken egg or goose egg.

6. Fish is also another useful thing into your daily menu, try to eat it at least two times per week.

7. Include fruits, but be aware that there is a lot of sugar in them, especially in tropical fruits, take you look mostly at berries. Fruits contain fructose which is not that good for the liver. But it is not that strict rule, so you can sometimes include apple, avocado, blackberries, peaches, plums, blueberries, lemon, watermelon, pineapple, oranges into your menu.

8. Try to include nuts into your daily menu, especially almonds, pistachios, cashews, hazelnuts etc.

9. Kefir, sour cream, different yogurts are allowed, they are very useful for the health in general.

10. It is better lower the intake of nuts, fruits to nearly 50 – 70 grams per day. If you wish to loose weight rapidly.

11. Eat if only you are hungry and every three hours.

12. Spare enough time for sleep it is better to make a regime for yourself, for instance sleep from ten pm till seven am the least.

13. Try to take not very hard exercise two times per week. Combine your exercise program, with daily rest.

14. Include vitamin D in your menu as it is one more important ingredient. Iodine is another important ingredient into your daily menu. You can take this vitamin from seaweeds, they are really reach for it.

15. You are free to eat leafy greens, like: spinach, iceberg lettuce, kale etc.

16. You can afford yourself even Dark Chocolate. It is necessary to find the dark chocolate of at least 70% - 80% cacao.

17. It is also possible to enjoy one glass of red wine per day.

18. You should drink at least one and a half liters of water per day.

19. It is necessary to mention some foods you should avoid to stay slim and healthy according to the rules of paleo diet. Natural carbs: Potatoes, Rice, milk , but dairy is allowed especially if you feel that it is necessary for your organs of digestion.

20. The most beautiful thing is that you do not have to limit your daily intake of food. But of course it is better to eat till the moment when you can feel that you are not hungry anymore, and not till when you are totally full.

21. Try to get outside to get sunshine as the more vitamin D you get the better for your health, but do not get burned!

22. Obtain a crock pot, as it is the best method to prepare paleo meals.

23. Do not hurry to see the results. Paleo diet is not a one day diet, it takes time, but it gives results as well.

24. Lower the intake of salt as it is not a good thing to your kidneys. It is worth mentioning, when you remove a lot of "negative foods" from your menu you will understand that it is totally ok to eat without salt and sugar, or cook with the help of crock pot and the food tastes better, much better.

25. You can enjoy of all sort of animal organs like: tongue, kidney liver and marrow.

26. You can also enjoy eating different sea food things like: shrimps, scallops, herring, shark and much more.

27. It is also allowed to include different sorts of mushrooms. They are totally allowed.

28. You can use a lot of substitution to feel yourself satisfied with what you it, there are some of them listed below:
    - Sea salt instead of iodized salt.
    - Homemade paleo bread, instead of bread you can buy at the market.
    - Cauliflower instead of rice and potatoes.

29. Remember! All sorts of fruit juices are also very rich in fructose so it is better to stay away from them. These are

- Apple juice
- Orange juice
- Grape juice
- Strawberry juice
- Mango juice

30. It is also necessary to stay away from snacks. These are all sorts of chips, cookies, different pastries etc.

31. Also remove alcohol and energy drink from your list if you wish to stay healthy and lose your extra weight.

Chapter 2

IN THIS CHAPTER I WOULD LIKE TO GIVE YOU A VERY IMPORTANT INFORMATION AS FOR YOUR DAILY MENU, WHICH WILL HELP YOU TO START YOUR PALEO DIET EASILY. SO LETS BEGIN!

**For breakfast**:

The best and the healthiest thing will be omelet with some onion, broccoli or mushrooms. You can also add chicken or turkey.

**For Lunch:**

The best thing is to prepare a big bowl with vegetables like radish, spinach, cucumbers, carrot, you can also add almonds or walnuts. You are welcome to add such sorts of meat as chicken, turkey, beef to your plate or you can add something from fish like shrimp, tuna, salmon etc.

**For Dinner:**

It is possible to make a spaghetti squash instead of pasta recipe with meatballs, or also different sorts of seafood or fresh food with broccoli, or vegetables a great idea for paleo dinner.

# Paleo Diet for Beginners:

80 Healthy Paleo Recipes and 31 Proven Steps to Loose Weight

You can take berries for your dessert

# Paleo Diet for Beginners:

80 Healthy Paleo Recipes and 31 Proven Steps to Loose Weight

15 yummy paleo recipes for every day.

Breakfast recipes:

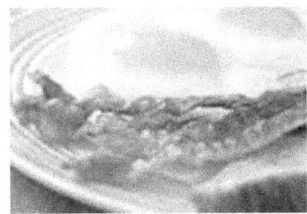

# 1.Becon and egg Paradise

**Ingredients:**

3 - 6 eggs

3 slices of cut bacon

2 cups of spinach chopped

A bit of salt and pepper

**Instructions:**

Heat your oven to 350F

Mix the eggs in a bowl

# Paleo Diet for Beginners:

### 80 Healthy Paleo Recipes and 31 Proven Steps to Loose Weight

Cook the becon in a skillet

Add a spinach to this skillet and cook for 10 more minutes

Add eggs into this skillet and add a bit of salt and pepper.

Bake for 15 more minutes

# Paleo Diet for Beginners:

80 Healthy Paleo Recipes and 31 Proven Steps to Loose Weight

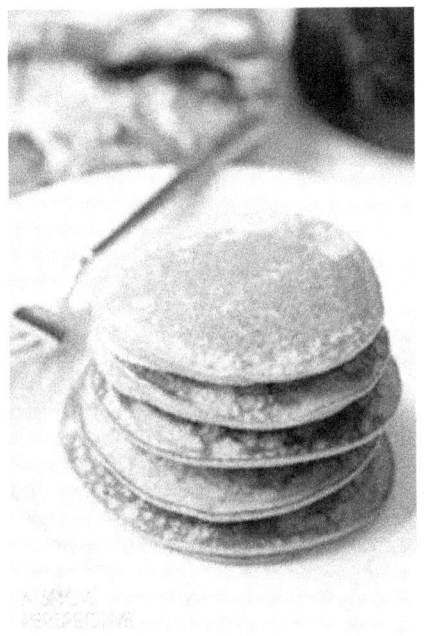

## 2. Perfect Paleo Pancakes (nut-free)

**Ingredients:**

4 Eggs

Half of a cup of coconut flour

1table spoon of honey

1 table spoon of vinegar

a half of a spoon of baking soda

a bit of a salt

1 table spoon of vanilla

**Instructuions:**

1. Put all the dry pancake ingredients in a bowl. Whip in all the liquid ingredients (do not add the coconut milk).
2. Gradually add the coconut milk. You will need to add as much coconut milk as you need until you see the preferable consistency.
3. Preheat a consistency and coat with grease with coconut oil.
4. Pour a spoon of a pancake batter onto the griddle. Make the pancakes about 3-4 inches in diameter as it will be easier to operate them. Bake for 2-3 minutes, then turn them on another side for an additional 1-2 minutes.
5. Take away from a pan and serve with your chosen syrup.

Enjoy your breakfast.

# Paleo Diet for Beginners:

80 Healthy Paleo Recipes and 31 Proven Steps to Loose Weight

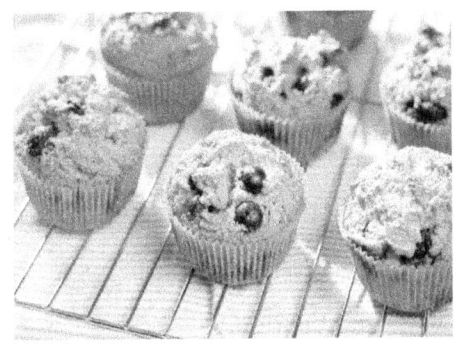

## 3. Paleo Blueberry Muffin

**Ingredients:**

1 cup of almond flour

A bit of soda

A bit of salt on your taste

1 egg

2 tbsp of honey

A half of a cup of fresh blueberries

A half of a cup of coconut milk

2 tbsp of coconut oil

# Paleo Diet for Beginners:

80 Healthy Paleo Recipes and 31 Proven Steps to Loose Weight

## Instructions:

1. Heat the oven to 350°F.
2. Mix all together salt, baking soda and almond flour
3. Whip all together the honey, coconut milk, coconut oil, and egg.
4. Then mix the wet and the dry ingredients together, but not that much.
5. Add blueberries into the dough.
6. Add the prepared dough into the muffin tin and bake
7. Bake until a toothpick inserted into the center comes out clean, about 20-25 minutes
8. Set pan over a wire rack to cool. Wait until muffins are completely cool before removing from the paper liners.

Recipe makes 6 muffins. Store in an airtight container in the refrigerator.

# Paleo Diet for Beginners:

80 Healthy Paleo Recipes and 31 Proven Steps to Loose Weight

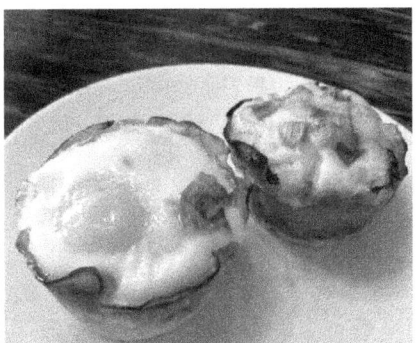

## 4. Paleo Breakfast: Baked Eggs in Ham Cups

**Ingredients:**

Eggs

Ham or Turkey

**Instructions:**

1. Heat the oven to 400°F.

2. Grease your muffin pan.

3. Slice the ham and put it into the muffin cup, one or two slices is enough for each cup.

4. You can scramble your eggs or even whip them or you can just put the whole egg into the muffin cup. (Optional) If you do wish to make scrambled eggs you can also add there different ingredients, like mushrooms, onion, different greens and spinach.

5. Preheat the oven ti 400°F , put the muffin pan in to the oven and bake for 15 – 20 more minutes

# Paleo Diet for Beginners:

80 Healthy Paleo Recipes and 31 Proven Steps to Loose Weight

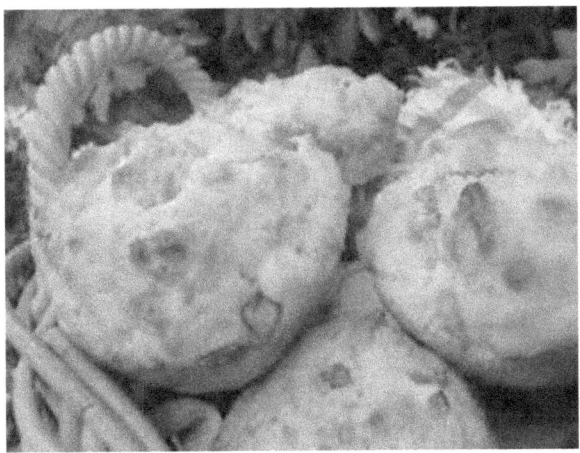

## 5. Avocado & Bacon Muffins

**Ingredients:**

1 onion

4 eggs

6 -7 slices of bacon

2 cups avocado

one and a half of a cup of coconut flour

a half of a tea spoon of baking soda

salt & pepper

1 cup of coconut milk

# Paleo Diet for Beginners:

80 Healthy Paleo Recipes and 31 Proven Steps to Loose Weight

**Instructions:**

1. Heat the oven to 175 degrees Celsius (350F)

2. Grease 12 muffin pans with oil. (melt it before)

3. Finely chop onion and bacon.

4. Brown in a fry pan.

5. Mix the avocado and eggs very good.

6. Stir in the milk.

7. Add coconut flour, salt, pepper and baking soda and stir it all well

8. Fold through three quarters of the cooked bacon and onion mixture.

9. Put this into the muffin pans.

10. Put on the top bacon and onion.

11. Bake in the oven for approximately 20 25 minutes.

12. Cool before taking the muffins out.

13. Enjoy your breakfast.

# Paleo Diet for Beginners:

80 Healthy Paleo Recipes and 31 Proven Steps to Loose Weight

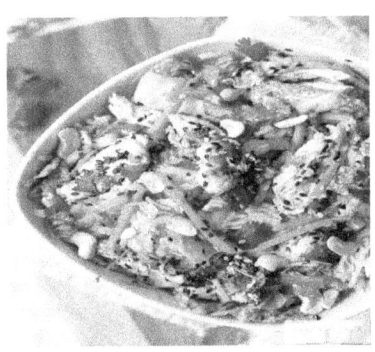

## 6.Super Paleo Chinese Chicken Salad

**Ingredients:**

1 carrot

1 large Napa Cabbage, it is necessary to chop it into slices.

1 chicken, sliced into thin peaces.

A half of a cup chopped cilantro

2 tablespoons of black sesame seeds and 2 table spoons of white sesame seeds

1/4 cup of gluten free soy sauce, I prefer Tamari.

1/4 cup white wine vinegar

3 table spoons of a minced ginger

3 table spoons of olive oil

1 table spoon of toasted sesame oil

1 table spoon of Spicy Chili Oil

Some sea salt on your taste

Some chopped green onions

**For the dressing:**

In a small bowl with lid add tamari sauce, vinegar, olive oil, hoisin sauce, toasted sesame oil, chili oil, sriracha, minced ginger, sea salt and chopped green onions. Shake it all together. Set aside. Then add, chopped cabbage, sliced carrot, cilantro, sesame seeds, cashews, sliced chicken, and dressing into a large plastic bowl, shake until well enough. Add more dressing if needed.

# Paleo Diet for Beginners:

80 Healthy Paleo Recipes and 31 Proven Steps to Loose Weight

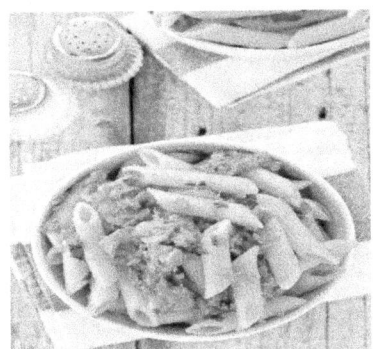

## 7. Spicy Tuna and Tomato

**Ingredients:**

1 cup of tuna

1 red onion, chopped

1 small red chilli, chopped as well

1 peace of garlic

1 egg

2 Tbsp of tomato paste

1 Tbsp of coconut flour

# Paleo Diet for Beginners:

## 80 Healthy Paleo Recipes and 31 Proven Steps to Loose Weight

Salt and pepper on your taste

You can also add:

Lettuce

Avocado

Extra chilli, if you wish it to be hot


**Instructions:**

1 – Pre-heat your oven to 350'F

2 – Put a parchment paper on a baking tray and set aside for now.

3 – Put all the burger ingredients into a bowl and stir all them well

4. Make with your hands bolls using this tuna mixture. Place all of them into the baking sheet

5 – Place in the oven and cook approximately for 5-10 mins, until they are cooked enough.

6 – To serve, place these cute balls on a lettuce leaf (or 2) put some fresh sliced avocado on top, and sprinkle over some fresh coriander and some slices of chilli.

Enjoy your meal!

# Paleo Diet for Beginners:

80 Healthy Paleo Recipes and 31 Proven Steps to Loose Weight

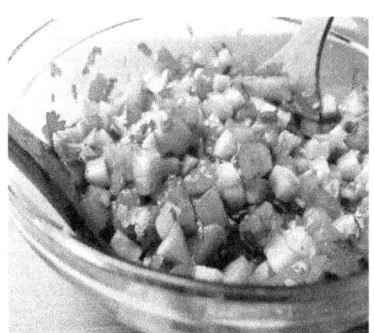

## 8. Cucumber and Tomato Salad

**Ingredients:**

one clove Garlic

one cup of Olives

one tablespoon of fresh Basil, (it is necessary to slice it very thin)

one table spoon of Fresh Oregano, (it is necessary to chop it)

two cups of Cucumber, sliced or chopped.

Two cups of Grape Tomatoes

Two table spoons of Balsamic Vinegar

Two table spoons of Extra Virgin Olive Oil

One table spoon of Black Pepper

**Instructions:**

# Paleo Diet for Beginners:

80 Healthy Paleo Recipes and 31 Proven Steps to Loose Weight

1. Rinse, then slice or chop your cucumbers.
2. Rinse grape tomatoes, cut them in half.
3. Thinly slice basil, cut oregano, mince garlic.
4. Mix everything with the kalamata olives in a bowl, sprinkle with olive oil and balsamic vinegar, and add a bit of black pepper.

# Paleo Diet for Beginners:

80 Healthy Paleo Recipes and 31 Proven Steps to Loose Weight

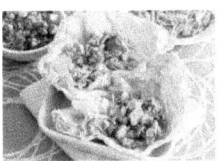

# 9.Chicken and avocado Lettuce Wraps

**Ingredients:**

One cup cooked and sliced Chicken, Boneless Breasts

One and a half cup of mashed avocado, peel the coat before mashing.
one tbsp. of juice Lemon

one tbsp. of juice Lime

two tbsp. of Yogurt

two tbsp of choped Cilantro

Salt on your taste

Black Pepper on your taste

Serving Day Ingredients

One cup of grape tomatoes

## Instructions:

1. Chop chicken breast
2. Mash avocado, lemon juice, lime juice, and yogurt in a bowl and stir well, until it becomes creamy!
3. Add salt, pepper and cilantro to the chopped chicken, according to your taste.
4. Spoon into lettuce wraps, put tomatoes on top, and serve.

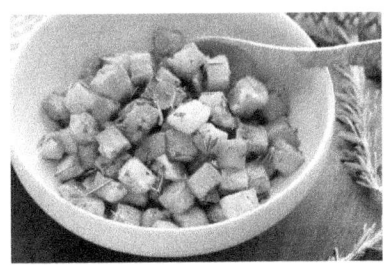

## 10.Swett Potato

**Ingredients:**

2 Medium sweet potatoes chopped into small cubes

3 tbsp of coconut oil

Sea salt

**Instructions:**

1. Boil water in a medium pot
2. Chop sweet potato into cubes

3. Put the sweet potato into the boiling water for around five minutes and take It away when it becomes slightly softened.

4. Drain and dry the sweet potatoes

5. Heat up the coconut oil in the large skillet, make the heat medium.

6. Toss in the sweet potatoes cubes and let them cook well for approximately six or seven minutes. Continue doing it until they are nice and brown. Sprinkle with sea salt according to your taste. Your sweet potatoes will be yummy, crispy and goldy brown if you let them cook well enough.

ENJOY YOUR MEAL!

DINNER RECIPES

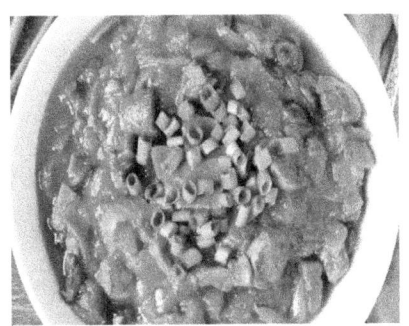

## 11.Paleo Pizza Soup

**Ingredients:**

10-12 chicken sausage, slice them

4 – 5 uncured pepperoni,

5-7 roasted tomatoes

1 medium size onion,

10-15 mushrooms, slice them

1 can of black olives, slice them

1 tbsp of dried oregano

1 tsp of garlic powder

Salt to taste

**Instructions:**

1. Put the sausage, pepperoni, marinara, tomatoes, onion, mushrooms, olives, oregano, garlic powder, and salt into the pan
2. Cook for about 30 minutes. It is considered to be ready when onions and mushrooms have softened.
3. Add more salt if needed.
4. Serve hot.
5. Enjoy this delicious meal.

# Paleo Diet for Beginners:

## 80 Healthy Paleo Recipes and 31 Proven Steps to Loose Weight

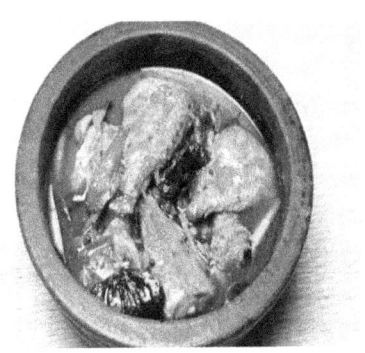

## 12.Quick and Easy Fish Curry

**Ingredients:**

2 Tbsp of coconut oil

1 onion,

3 cloves of garlic, chopped or mashed

2 Tbsp of ginger

2 tsp of curry powder

10 - 15 curry leaves

400ml of coconut milk

2 tomatoes, chopp them

# Paleo Diet for Beginners:

## 80 Healthy Paleo Recipes and 31 Proven Steps to Loose Weight

Sea salt on your taste

600g of white fish, cut into peaces

Juice of a lime on your taste

Large handful leaves of coriander

**Instructions:**

1. Melt the coconut oil in the pan.

2. Add sliced onion there and make it brown

3. Than add the garlic and ginger and cook for approximately one minute.

4. Add the turmeric, curry leaves and do not forget about the curry powder.

5. Continue to cook during one minute, then gradually stir in the coconut milk.

6. Simmer it.

7. Add the chopped tomato and simmer for additional five minutes until the tomato become soft.

8. Add the fish, add some salt on your taste and wait until the fish is cooked.

9. Add coriander and lime juice and stir it all well.

10. It is a very delicious with rice

# Paleo Diet for Beginners:

80 Healthy Paleo Recipes and 31 Proven Steps to Loose Weight

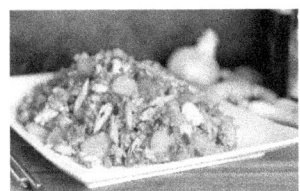

# 13.Paleo Pineapple Fried Rice

**Ingredients:**

Three table spoons of avocado oil

two cups of fresh pineapple, cut for the slices

one red bell pepper

four small carrots

two cloves garlic, minced

a bit of green onions, thinly sliced

four eggs

**Sauce:**

¼ cup coconut aminos

2 tsp of chili paste

# Paleo Diet for Beginners:

80 Healthy Paleo Recipes and 31 Proven Steps to Loose Weight

**As a final step:**

one cup of roasted cashew pieces

Sea salt on your taste

**Instructions:**

1. Prepare all your ingredients, wash and cut them
2. Take away the core with its seeds from the bell pepper and cut it thoroughly.
3. Peel the carrots and cut it into cubes.
4. Grate the cauliflower.
5. Crack the eggs into a plastic bowl and mix them with the fork or whatever.
6. Put together the coconut aminos and chili paste in a bowl and set it aside.
7. After you have prepared everything, preheat your pan
8. Add one tbsp of the avocado oil to the frying pan and also add the pineapple chunks to create the tasty and caramelized edges. Then take away the pineapples and put it into the separate bowl, until you prepare the rice. After add the green onions and cauliflower. It is necessary to cook it for about several minutes to make the cauliflower soft.
9. Then add all the veggies into the pan; pepper, garlic, carrots and make them crispy.
10. Add the sauce to the pan and let it to prepare for several more minutes until the sauce is gone and mix everything well.
11. Take away the fried rice from the heat and join it to cashews and caramelized pineapple. Add some sea salt if necessary.
12. It tastes simply amazing both hot and taken from the refrigerator.

# Paleo Diet for Beginners:

80 Healthy Paleo Recipes and 31 Proven Steps to Loose Weight

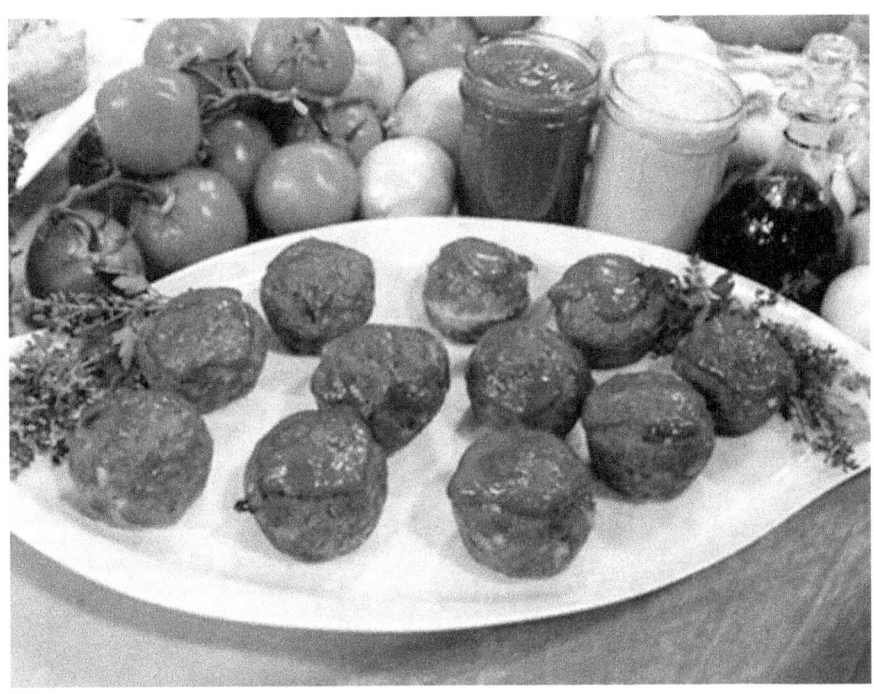

## 14. Paleo Mini Meatloaves

**Ingredients:**

two pounds of meat – it is better to mix beef with pork or veal

chopped spinach, the amount on your preference

one or two teaspoons oil

one medium onion,

ten - fifteen mushrooms, finely diced

# Paleo Diet for Beginners:

80 Healthy Paleo Recipes and 31 Proven Steps to Loose Weight

two grated carrots,

four eggs,

1/3 cup coconut flour

two tsp of salt

two tsp of pepper

two tsp of onion powder

one tsp of garlic powder

one tsp of dried thyme and a bit of grated nutmeg.

## Instructions:

1. Preheat oven to **375 degrees F**
2. Prepare spinach and set aside.
3. Preheat a pan add the oil and add there onions, mushrooms. Cook everything until the onion become translucent and some water is gone. Than you can set this pan aside. Place the ground meat in a large bowl, add the spinach, carrots, mushroom/onion mixture, beaten eggs, coconut flour and all the spices. Mix everything, but not that much, just to make all the ingredients well – organized.
4. Add this mixture into muffin tins. It is better to grease the tins.
5. Cook for 20-25 minutes until total preparation.
6. This dish is better to serve hot.

# Paleo Diet for Beginners:

80 Healthy Paleo Recipes and 31 Proven Steps to Loose Weight

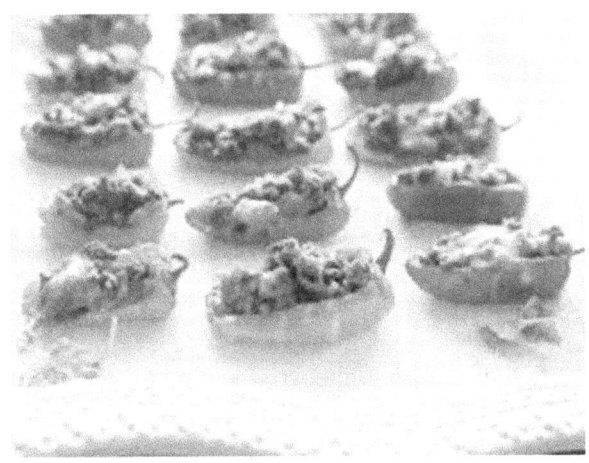

## 15. Stuffed Baby Sweet Peppers

**Ingredients:**

Fifteen - twenty mini sweet peppers

Six ounces of goat cheese

A half of a cup of ricotta cheese

One tea spoon of garlic powder

A bit of pepper powder

Salt to your taste

**Instructions:**

1. Preheat oven to 375F. Lean baking sheet with foil.

2. Wash the peppers and cut in half lengthwise. Remove all the seeds

3. Than mash together the goat cheese, the ricotta, and the seasonings well.

4. Snip the corner off of a small ziploc bag and put cheese mixture into this bag. Squeeze the bag and pipe the cheese into the pepper halves.

5. Put the peppers on the baking sheet and cook it for about 5-6 minutes until nicely browned. It is possible to prepare this delicious thing on the grill as well.

6. Enjoy!

Some more Paleo Recipes

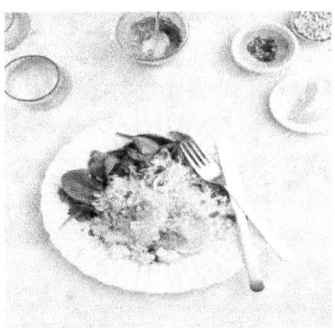

## 16. Creamy Lemon Basil Spaghetti Squash

**Ingredients:**

One Avocado (a half of a cup mashed)

six garlic cloves

one cup fresh basil leaves

one tbsp lemon zest

one third of a cup lemon juice

# Paleo Diet for Beginners:

80 Healthy Paleo Recipes and 31 Proven Steps to Loose Weight

two tbsp. of olive oil

if you wish you can add cayenne pepper on your taste

a half of tsp black pepper

a sea salt on your taste

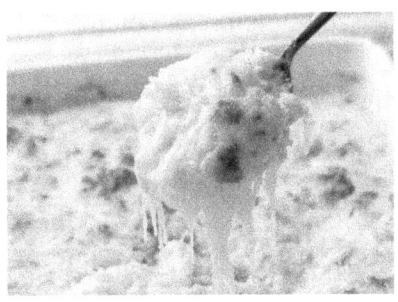

# 17. Spaghetti Squash

## Ingredients:

1. two tsp olive oil
2. three cups spaghetti squash, cooked
3. one cup of chopped kale
4. 10-15 cherry tomatoes
5. A half of tsp black pepper
6. sea salt on your taste

# Paleo Diet for Beginners:

80 Healthy Paleo Recipes and 31 Proven Steps to Loose Weight

**Instructions:**

1. Mix all the sauce ingredients into blender. Puree them thoroughly

2. Heat the pan and add the olive oil. When the oil is hot add the tomatoes and sauté about two minutes.

3. Add the other ingredients and sauté approximately five minutes. Add about a half of a cup of the sauce and mix thoroughly.

4. Bon appetite!!!

# Paleo Diet for Beginners:

80 Healthy Paleo Recipes and 31 Proven Steps to Loose Weight

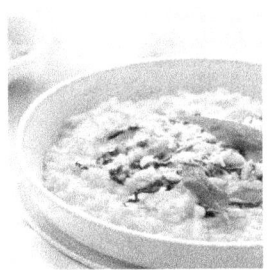

## 18. Butternut Squash Risotto

**Ingredients:**

1½ pounds butternut squash, peeled and cubed (about 4 cups)

1 tablespoon solid cooking fat

½ yellow onion, chopped

1 cup mushrooms, chopped

3 cloves garlic, minced

¼ cup sage, minced

½ teaspoon sea salt

1 teaspoon apple cider vinegar

¾ cup bone broth

# Paleo Diet for Beginners:

80 Healthy Paleo Recipes and 31 Proven Steps to Loose Weight

## Instructions:

1. Place half of the chopped butternut squash into a food processor and pulse for 20 seconds, until the squash is the consistency of rice. Don't over process here!

2. Heat the solid cooking fat in the bottom of a large skillet or heavy-bottomed pot on medium heat. When the fat has melted and the pan is hot, add the onions and mushrooms. Cook, stirring, until the onions are translucent, about 5 minutes. Add the garlic, sage, and sea salt, and cook for another 2 minutes, just until fragrant.

3. Add the apple cider vinegar and scrape away anything that has stuck to the bottom of the pan. Add the processed squash and bone broth to the pan, stirring to incorporate. Cook for 12-15 minutes on medium heat uncovered, stirring occasionally, until the liquid has absorbed and the squash is fully cooked.

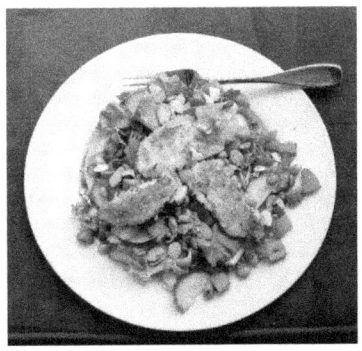

## 19. Coconut Crusted Chicken Salad

**Ingredients:**

2 tbsp Coconut flour

2 tbsp Unsweetened flaked coconut

2 Chicken fillets

1 Egg (beaten)

2 cups Spring mix salad greens

3 tbsp Apple cider vinegar

1 tsp Honey

# Paleo Diet for Beginners:

80 Healthy Paleo Recipes and 31 Proven Steps to Loose Weight

3 tbsp olive oil

2 tbsp Coconut oil

Salt and pepper (to taste)

## Instructions:

1. Create a breading/dredging station with three plates or shallow bowls.
2. Add the coconut flour to one, the the egg to the second plate and the flaked coconut to the third.
3. Heat the coconut oil in a skillet over medium-high heat.
4. Dredge each chicken fillet in the coconut flour first, followed by the egg, coating each evenly. Then the flaked coconut. Be sure the fillet is coated well.
5. Place each fillet into the hot skillet. Cook on each side, about 5 minutes. Until the chicken is golden in color and cooked through.
6. Add the apple cider vinegar and honey to a bowl. Whisk to combine. Continue to whisk while drizzling in the olive oil until well combined and becomes creamy. Season with salt and pepper.
7. Place the spring mix in a mixing bowl. Drizzle the dressing over and toss to coat. Reserve ½ to serving.
8. Plate the spring mix evenly then serve the chicken on top. Serve with additional dressing on the side. Season with salt and pepper, to taste.

# Paleo Diet for Beginners:

80 Healthy Paleo Recipes and 31 Proven Steps to Loose Weight

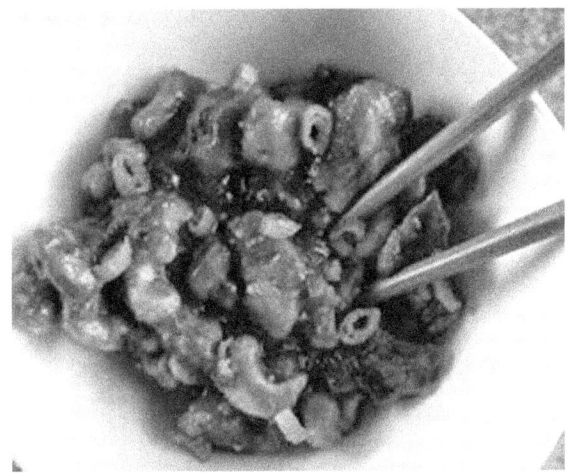

# 20. Paleo Crock Pot Cashew Chicken

**Ingredients:**

1/4 cup arrowroot starch

1/2 tsp. black pepper

2 lbs. chicken thighs, cut into bite-size pieces

1 tbs. coconut oil

3 tbs. coconut aminos

2 tbs. rice wine vinegar

2 tbs. organic ketchup (tomato paste would work also)

1/2-1 tbs. palm sugar

80 Healthy Paleo Recipes and 31 Proven Steps to Loose Weight

2 minced garlic cloves

1/2 tsp. minced fresh ginger

1/4-1/2 red pepper flakes

1/2 cup raw cashews

**Instructions:**

Place starch and black pepper in a large Ziploc bag. Add chicken pieces and seal; toss to thoroughly coat meat.

Melt coconut oil in a large skillet or wok. Add chicken and cook for about 5 minutes until brown on all sides. Remove and add to crock pot.

Mix coconut aminos through red pepper flakes in a small bowl. Pour mixture over chicken and toss to coat. Put lid on crock pot and cook on low for 3-4 hours.

Stir cashews into chicken and sauce before serving.

# Paleo Diet for Beginners:

80 Healthy Paleo Recipes and 31 Proven Steps to Loose Weight

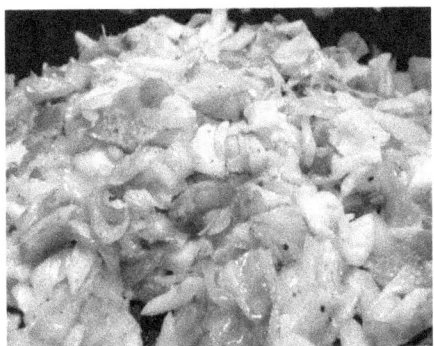

# 21. Fried Cabbage with Bacon, Onion, and Garlic

**Ingredients:**

Six slices of chopped becon

one large onion

two cloves of garlic

One cabbage

Salt on your taste

Pepper on your taste

A half of a teaspoon of onion powder

A half of a tea spoon of garlic powder

# Paleo Diet for Beginners:

80 Healthy Paleo Recipes and 31 Proven Steps to Loose Weight

**Instructions:**

1. Put the bacon in a large stockpot and cook it until it becomes crispy. It should take you about ten minutes. Add the garlic and onion. cook until the onion caramelizes; about ten minutes. Then Stir in the cabbage and continue to cook and stir for another 10 minutes. Add salt, pepper, onion powder, paprika and garlic powder. After all simmer for about 30 minutes more.

# Paleo Diet for Beginners:

80 Healthy Paleo Recipes and 31 Proven Steps to Loose Weight

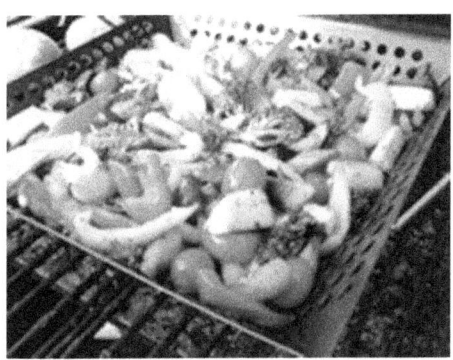

## 22. Roasted Tasty Vegetable Medley

**Ingredients:**

2 tbsp olive oil

One yam, peeled and cut into pieces.

One parsnip, peeled and cut into pieces.

One carrot

One zucchini, cut into pieces

One bunch of a fresh asparagus, also cut into pieces

# Paleo Diet for Beginners:

80 Healthy Paleo Recipes and 31 Proven Steps to Loose Weight

Two cloves of a minced garlic

Fresh basil, on your taste

Pepper on your taste

**Instructions:**

1. Heat the oven and grease the baking sheet with olive oil.
2. Put the yams, parsnips, and carrots onto the baking sheets. Bake in the oven for 30 minutes, after put the zucchini and asparagus, and sprinkle with the 1 tablespoon of olive oil. Proceed baking until all of the vegetables are cooked, about 30 minutes more. Then remove from the oven, and allow to cool.
3. Toss the roasted peppers with the garlic, basil, salt, and pepper in a large bowl. Add the roasted vegetables, and mix everything well.

# Paleo Diet for Beginners:

80 Healthy Paleo Recipes and 31 Proven Steps to Loose Weight

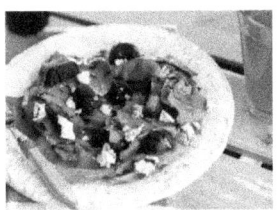

## 23. Delicious Beet Greens

**Ingredients:**

Two bunches beet greens

One table spoon of olive oil

Two cloves of garlic minced

Red pepper on your taste

Salt and pepper on your taste

Two lemons, cut into four slices

# Paleo Diet for Beginners:

80 Healthy Paleo Recipes and 31 Proven Steps to Loose Weight

**Instructions:**

1. Put water into a pot let it to boil and salt it. Add the beet greens and cook them until they become tender. It will take you about two minutes. Drain beet greens then immerse with the ice water.

2. Bring a large pot of lightly salted water to a boil. Add the beet greens, and cook uncovered until tender, about 2 minutes. Drain in a colander, then immediately immerse in ice water for several minutes. Then chop the greens.

3. Heat the olive oil. Stir in the garlic and red pepper; cook and stir for one minute. Add salt and pepper. Cook until greens are hot; serve with lemon.

# Paleo Diet for Beginners:

80 Healthy Paleo Recipes and 31 Proven Steps to Loose Weight

## Paleo Breakfast Recipes

## 24. ALMOND FLOUR PANCAKES

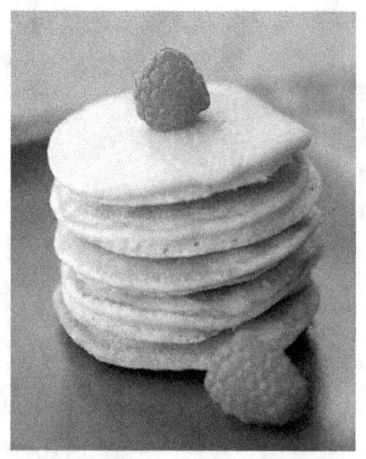

**Ingredients:**

one and a half cup of almond flour

one and a half cup of apple sauce, no sugar

one tbsp. of coconut flour

two large eggs

less than a half of a cup of a water

less than a half of tsp of nutmeg

less than a half of tsp of sea salt

one tsp of coconut oil

half of a cup of fresh berries

# Paleo Diet for Beginners:

80 Healthy Paleo Recipes and 31 Proven Steps to Loose Weight

**Instructions:**

1.Put all the ingredients into a bowl, like: almond flour, applesauce, coconut flour, eggs, water, nutmeg and sea salt.

2. Stir all this together with a fork.

3. Heat the frying pan with coconut oil.

4. Add one fourth of a batter into the pan

5. Flip like a usual pancake when you can see the bubbles and prepare for one more minute.

6. Add some oil and repeat with the remaining batter.

7. Put some fresh berries on the top.

## 25. APPLE CINNAMON MUFFINS

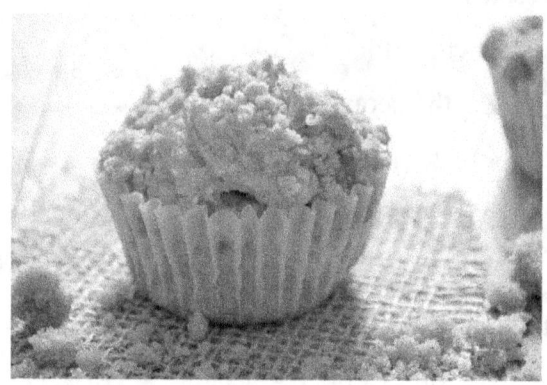

**Ingredients:**

Two small apples cored and diced

One tbsp. of lemon juice

Five large eggs

 A half of a cup of coconut flour

Two tablespoons of cinnamon

A bit of ground nutmeg

One tbsp. of baking soda

Four tsp of melted coconut oil

A bit of a sea salt

One package of paper muffin liners

# Paleo Diet for Beginners:

80 Healthy Paleo Recipes and 31 Proven Steps to Loose Weight

**Instructions:**

1. Preheat the oven, sprinkle a muffin tin with cooking spray or it is possible just to put paper liners.

2. Put all the apples into the saucepan and cover. It is necessary to add enough water so it will cover almost the half. Wait until it boils and later reduce heat and let it simmer for 10 minutes. You will be sure everything is ready when apples are broken down. Make everything smooth with the help of a blender.

3. Let the apples to cool, when everything is ready, add other ingredients to the blender and puree till the thick batter.

4. Add butter into your muffin tin

5. Bake approximately 15 -18 minutes until muffins get browned. Let them cool before taking out from the pan.

## 26. BANANA TAPIOCA CREPES

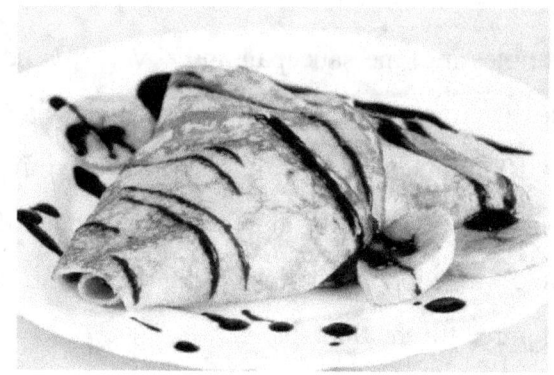

**Ingredients:**

Seven large eggs

Five large bananas

One can of coconut milk

One tsp of sea salt

Two and a half cups of starch or tapioca flour.

**Instructions:**

1. Put all the ingredients together and make a soupy butter
2. Preheat the pan
3. When the pan becomes hot add thin layer of batter
4. Cook until both sides are lightly browned.
5. These things are great for wrapping meat and veggies.

## 27. BERRY COCONUT CHIA SMOOTHIE

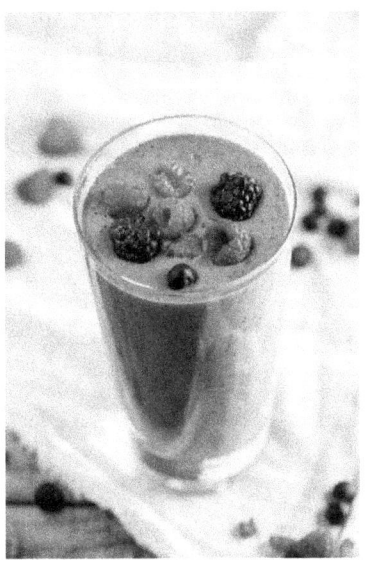

**Ingredients :**

One medium banana

Two tbsp. of chia seeds

Two cups of spinach baby

One tsp of coconut oil

One and a hald maybe even less of coconut milk, full fat

One cup of frozen berries

One tablespoon of coconut flakes, if you wish to garnish your dish

One tablespoon of chia seeds if you wish to garnish your dish

# Paleo Diet for Beginners:

## 80 Healthy Paleo Recipes and 31 Proven Steps to Loose Weight

**Instructions:**

Put all the stuff into the blan der and blend everything until smooth

## 28. CARROT BANANA MUFFINS

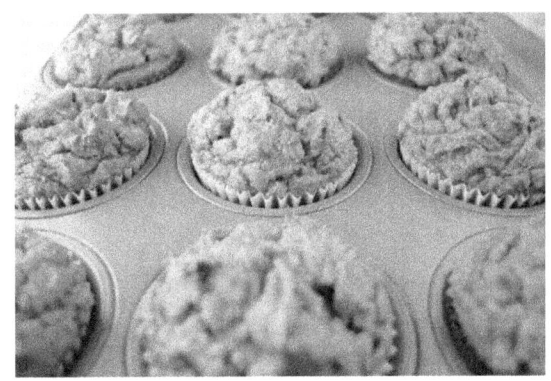

**Ingredients:**

Two cups of almond flour

Two teaspoons of baking soda

A half of a teaspoon of sea salt

Of tablespoon of cinnamon

One cup of dates

Three medium bananas

Three large eggs

One teaspoon of apple cider vinegar

One fourth of a cup of coconut oil melted

One and a half of a large carrot

A bit of walnuts finely chopped

And paper muffin liners

**Instructions:**

1. Heat the oven to 350 F.
2. Put together baking soda, salt and cinnamon in a bowl.
3. Add bananas, eggs, vinegar and oil in a food processor.
4. Combine everything plus add carrots and nuts
5. Put this prepared mixture into paper lined muffin tins.
6. Bake for about 30 minutes at 350 F

## 29. CHORIZO RICE WITH FRIED EGG

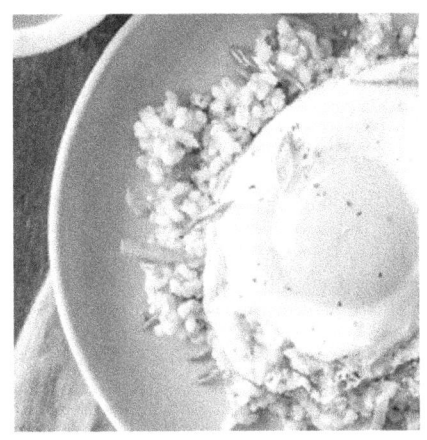

**Ingredients:**

One pound of ground chorizo

One half of cauliflower

One small onion, diced

One garlic clove , minced

Small bell paper, diced as well

Two eggs

Two tbsp. of a lard

A bit of salt on your taste

A bit of black pepper on your taste

# Paleo Diet for Beginners:

80 Healthy Paleo Recipes and 31 Proven Steps to Loose Weight

**Instructions:**

1. You can use a cheese grater to make your cauliflower of a rice like consistency.
2. Heat the pan and add one tbsp. of a lard. Add chorizo and cook for about 7 minutes.
3. Add onion, bell pepper and saute for 1 -2 minutes more.
4. Make the heat lower and add the riced cauliflower to the pan. Cook for another 5 minutes.
5. Also heat up one tablespoon of lard and fry eggs
6. Pile chorizo on a plate and put a fried egg ona top.
7. Garnish with green onions or cilantro if you wish!

## 30. COCONUT LIME PANCAKES

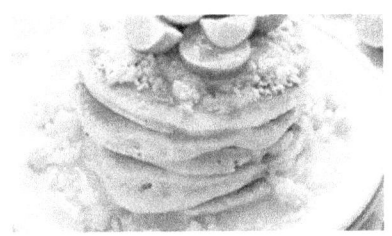

**Ingredients:**

One and a half cup of coconut, shredded

One and a half of a tsp of baking powder

Salt on your taste

One cup of almond flour

One lime, we need to use its juice

One egg

Two tbsp. of honey

One cup of coconut milk

A quarter of a cup of a water

Three tbsp. of coconut oil

Eight tbsp. of maple syrup

# Paleo Diet for Beginners:

80 Healthy Paleo Recipes and 31 Proven Steps to Loose Weight

## Instructions:

1. Heat the oven to 350 F. Put the coconut on the baking sheet and let it to brow for 4 – 5 minutes. After it gets brown put it to a blender jar.

2. Add the baking powder, lime, almond flour and sea salt to blender and blend it for about 5 seconds.

3. Add the lime juice, water, coconut milk, egg and honey in a bowl. Stir everything well. Add all this into the blender and blend all this stuff together. The batter should look pourable. If it is need add one or two tablespoons of water to make the batter thinner.

4. Hit an iron skillet to medium heat. Add the coconut oil and pour the batter into 3 – inch pancakes. Cook it until both sides will be browned.

# 31. EGG-FREE, GRAIN-FREE PUMPKIN ZUCCHINI MUFFINS

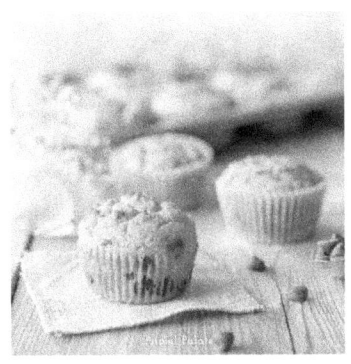

**Ingredients:**

Two tbsp. of flax seeds

Six tbsp. of water

One cup of almond flour

One and a half cups of coconut flour

One and a half cups of starch

Two teaspoons of baking soda

One tea spoon of sea salt (if you wish)

One tbsp. of cinnamon

One cup of dates

Two cups of pumpkin puree, organic

# Paleo Diet for Beginners:

80 Healthy Paleo Recipes and 31 Proven Steps to Loose Weight

One tsp of cider vinegar

One spoon of coconut oil

About 10 oz of frozen berries

Grated zucchini ¾ medium

A bit of sliced almonds

One package of paper muffin liners

**Instructions:**

1. Preheat oven to 350 F.
2. Mix together flax meal and water and let stay for about five minutes.
3. Mix almond flour, coconut flour, tapioca flour, sea salt, cinnamon, baking soda in a large bowl.
4. Put together dates, flax meal mixture, pumpkin, apple cider vinegar and coconut oil in food processor mix everything until dates are totally chopped. Fold into dry ingredients.
5. Add fold berries, nuts and berries into batter.
6. Put into paper lined muffin tins.
7. Bake them for about 20-25 minutes. Than you may turn of the oven and leave the muffins there.

## 32. FRIED EGGS WITH SWEET POTATO HASH

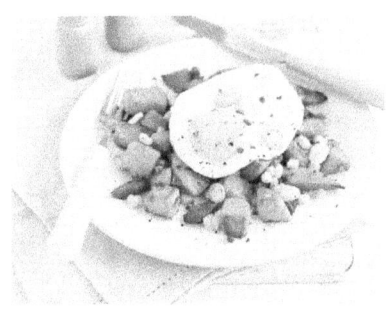

**Ingredients:**

One tbsp. Coconut oil

One sweet potato, diced into cubes

A half of an onion yellow, diced

Two sausage(s)

One bell pepper, diced

Two tablespoon(s) of water

Four large eggs

A half of a tsp black pepper

**Ingredients:**

1. Heat coconut oil in a large skillet
2. Satue onions and sweet potatoes for five minutes
3. Add sausages and cook all this together until all the ingredients get browned.
4. Add bell paper and water

5. Cook for about fifteen minutes until the potatoes are totally prepared, stir everything quit often.
6. During all this stuff are being prepared, fry eggs in coconut oil.
7. Season eggs with black pepper and serve all this over sweet potatoe.

## 33. LIVER SAUSAGE AND EGGS

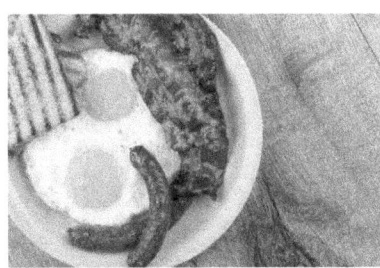

**Ingredients:**

Three forth pounds of pork

One and a half pound of beef

One forth pound of beef liver

One tsp of maple syrup

One tsp of sage

One and a half of dried thyme

One and a half of tsp of dried rosemary

One and a half of tsp of dried rosemary, sea salt, black pepper

Two tbsp. of olive oil

4 eggs.

**Instructions:**
1. Put together pork, beef, liver, maple syrup, seasonings, salt, pepper in a bowl. Mix everything thoroughly and form into two-inch patties.
2. Heat the olive oil in a skillet and cook these two patties until well browned. Remove the sausages, add the oil and fried the eggs. Serve with sausages.

## 34. PUMPKIN BREAD

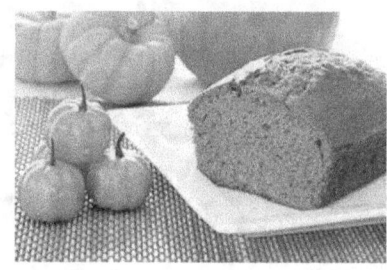

**Ingredients:**

One cup almond flour

a half of a cup of coconut flour

one  Tsp of cinnamon

½ tsp baking soda

½ tsp sea salt, fine grain

½  teaspoon pumpkin pie spice

$1/4$ teaspoon cloves


1 cup coconut sugar

½ cup pumpkin puree,

$1/3$ cup coconut oil, melted


3 tbsp coconut milk

1 whole vanilla beans

# Paleo Diet for Beginners:

80 Healthy Paleo Recipes and 31 Proven Steps to Loose Weight

4 large eggs

**Instructions:**

1. Preheat the oven to 325 F
2. Mix together the flours, cinnamon, salt, pumpkin pie spice, baking soda, cloves, and coconut sugar in the bowl of a large food processor. Then add the pumpkin puree, coconut oil, vanilla bean seeds, coconut milk, or extract, and eggs and process for 30 seconds.
3. Put the mixture to the parchment-lined loaf pan. Bake for 70 to 75 minutes. Let cool in the pan for fifteen minutes.

## 35. ROASTED PEPPER AND SAUSAGE OMELET

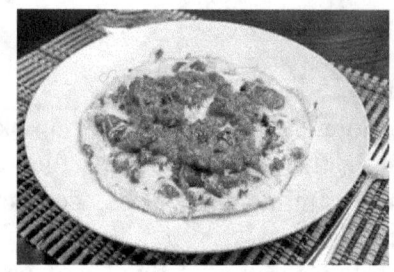

**Ingredients:**

One green chili or bell pepper.

Four eggs

A bit of a black pepper

2 tsp of coconut oil

One and a half pounds of Italian sausages or you can take beef, cook and slice it

2 tbsp of parsley

**Instructions:**

1. Put pepper into a pan with a heavy bottom. Make pepper`s skin blacken and blister. When the pepper is ready, remove from the pan and put it into plastic bag, you may add a few drops of water. Wait for 5 more minutes, remove from this bag, cut out seeds, peel the skin and dice.
2. After, beat eggs in a bowl and add black pepper.
3. Heat a skillet over medium heat. Add one tsp of coconut oil when hot.
4. Add half of the egg mixture to preheated pan. As the egg starts preparing, add another half of the remaining ingredients to one half of the pan.
5. When all is set, put half of the egg over the filling, and cook for another minute.
6. Do the same with the second omelet.

## 36. SUMMER VEGETABLE FRITTAT

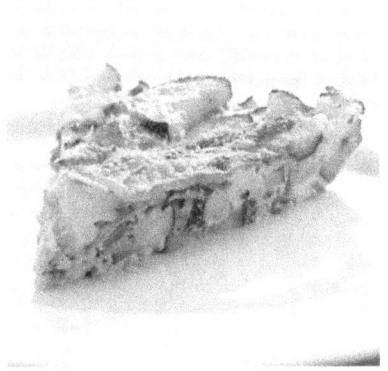

**Ingredients:**

One and a half tbsp. coconut oil or olive oil

One zucchini

One and a half bell pepper

One and a half onion, Diced

One tablespoon thyme

Sea salt on your taste

Black pepper on your taste

2 garlic cloves, minced

One tomato seeded

9 eggs

# Paleo Diet for Beginners:

80 Healthy Paleo Recipes and 31 Proven Steps to Loose Weight

**Instructions:**

1. Heat coconut oil in a oven over medium heat. Add zucchini, pepper, onion, and half of the sea salt, thyme, garlic and pepper.
2. Cover and cook until vegetables are done (it may take you five – seven minutes), stir from time to time.
3. Add tomato. Cook for five more minutes.
4. Mix eggs and salt and pepper.
5. Pour eggs over vegetable mixture and stir everything. Lower heat and cook fifteen more minutes.
6. Put on a plate, slice and serve.

## 37. WESTERN OMELET

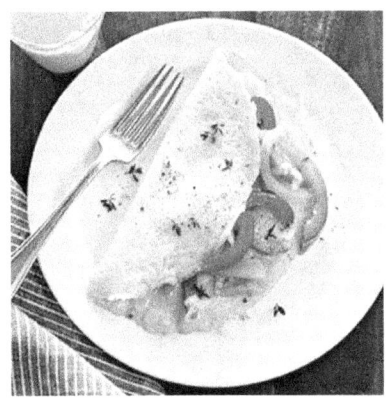

**Ingredients:**

Four large eggs

One tps of coconut oil

One and a half medium onion

One medium bell pepper

One tomato

One cup of spinach

One forth pounds of ham, cooked and diced

One forth tsp of salt

One forth tsp of black pepper

**Instructions:**

1. Wash and cut vegetables.
2. Put eggs into small pan and mix well.

3. Heat the skillet. When hot, add coconut oil to the pan.

4. Add half of the beaten eggs into the skillet. When the egg is almost cooked  make it pour all over the pan you    can help to do it with the fork.

5. Then, add half of the vegetables and ham to the omelet and proceed with the cooking process until the egg is almost prepared.

6. Using a spatula, fold the empty half over top of the ham and veggies. Cook for additional two minutes.

7. The second omelet make in the same way.

## 38. Veggie & Duck Egg Paleo Breakfast Muffins

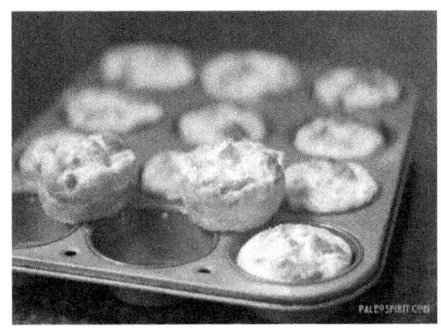

**Ingredients:**

1 and a half cups of eggplant, diced

Two diced mushrooms

Six tbsp. of tomato sauce

Six duck eggs

Savory leaves dried, according to your taste

Sea salt according to your taste as well

**Instructions:**

Preheat the oven to 350 F
Fill the muffin tin with parchment paper baking cups.
Fill these muffin cups with diced eggplant and mushrooms.
Add a teaspoon of homemade tomato sauce on top
Cracj a duck egg on top of the sauce
Put on the top of each muffin savory and some salt.
Put the muffin tin into the oven and cook for 15 minutes
Enjoy your meal!

## 39. Paleo Banana Nut Muffins

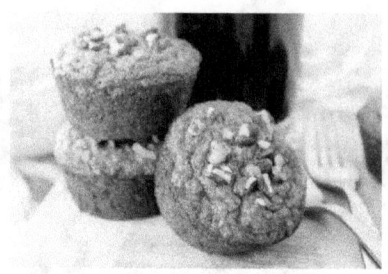

### Ingredients:

Two brown bananas
One and one forth cup of an almond flour
One forth cup of tapioca flour
One tsp of baking soda
Three eggs
A bit of raw walnuts
Two tbsp. of lard
A bit of sea salt on your taste
Two tbsp. of honey

### Instructions:

1. Heat the oven to 350 F
2. Peel the bananas and put them into the medium-sized bowl.
3. Also add the almond flour, tapioca flour and some baking soda to the bowl with bananas. Stir everything carefully.
4. Bake it for about thirty minutes
5. You can serve it either warm or cold.
6. Enjoy your meal.

## 40. Paleo Baked Avocado Fries Recipe

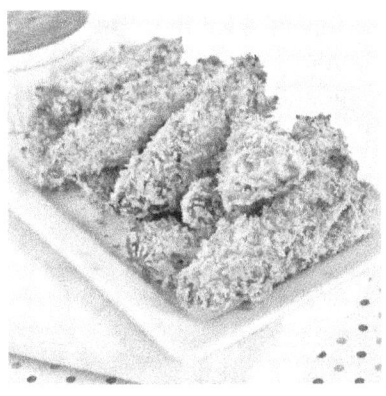

**Ingredients:**

two avocados

two tea spoon of garlic powder

one tea spoon of onion powder

1 tea spoon of paprika

sea salt on your taste

black pepper on your taste

about 50 g of tapioca flour

one egg

about 15 ml of water

a bitof a stone ground masterd

about 30 g of crushed pork rinds

# Paleo Diet for Beginners:

## 80 Healthy Paleo Recipes and 31 Proven Steps to Loose Weight

**Instructions:**

1. Heat the oven to 425°F
2. Cut the avocados in pieces. Divide each half into several slices, and set them aside.
3. You'll use three small bowls. Mix the arrowroot and half the seasonings into the first bowl. Beat the egg, water and mustard in the second bowl. Put the pork rinds and the other half of the seasonings into the third bowl.
4. After dip the avocado slices into the arrowroot, the next step is eggs, and after the pork rinds. Put everything on the baking sheet. Bake the avocado fries for about fifteen minutes, then turn and toss and bake for another 2 to 4 minutes.

## 41. Chocolate Collagen Protein Pancakes Recipe

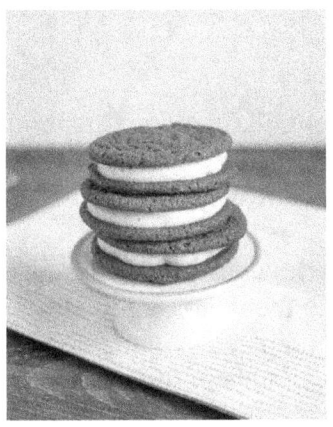

**Ingredients:**

One egg

Less than a half of almond milk

A half of a cup of a water

One table spoon of honey

Two table spoon of coconut oil

A bit of an almond meal

One forth cup of tapioca starch

Three tea spoon of baking powder

Three table spoon of cacao powder

One forth cup of collagen powder

A bit of salt on your taste

# Paleo Diet for Beginners:

## 80 Healthy Paleo Recipes and 31 Proven Steps to Loose Weight

You can also add some fresh fruits

You can put some honey on top if you like

**Instructions:**

Mix egg, water and almond milk in a bowl. After that add coconut oil and honey and mix everything thoroughly.

Mix almond meal, baking powder, salt, cocoa powder, tapioca starch and collagen in another bowl.

It is necessary to get a thick batter by joining together dry ingredients together with the wet ingredients by whisking them thoroughly.

Heat the coconut oil in the prepared skillet and put in the middle of it in the form of circle. When you see the bubbles on the top of the batter turn it over with the help of spatula and cook for another minute.

It is even more delicious to serve the pancakes with honey or fruits on the top.

## 42. Basic Chestnut Flour Crepes

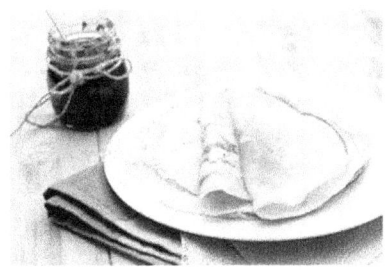

### Ingredients:

Two cups of chestnut flour

One cup of milk

one cup of water

one egg

one tbsp. of coconut oil

### Instructions:
1. Mix milk, water, and egg in a blender.
2. Add two hundred grams of chestnut flour in a blender
3. Add some melted butter it also can be oil.
4. Mix everything for five ten minutes.
5. Heat a skillet.
6. Pour the batter about one third of a cup into pan. Cook it until you see that the surface is no longer raw and you can see that the other side is already brown. If it is so than flip it on the other to make it golden.

**Snack Recipes**

## 43. ALMOND MUFFINS

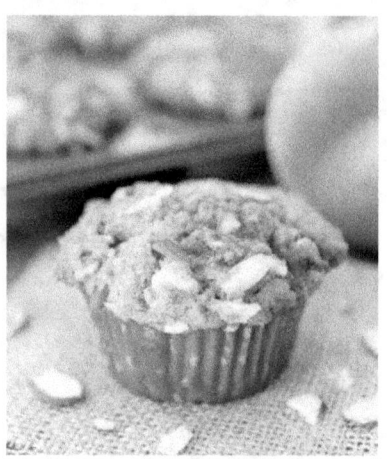

**Ingredients:**

One cup of almond butter

One cup of almonds

One cup of coconut milk

Two cups of coconut

Three large eggs

A bit of vanilla

Two tbsp. of honey (if you like it)

One package of muffin liners

# Paleo Diet for Beginners:

80 Healthy Paleo Recipes and 31 Proven Steps to Loose Weight

**Instructions:**

Heat the oven to 400F

Line a tin with the necessary paper

Mix together all the ingredients and put into the muffin tin.

Bake for about twenty minutes.

## 44. BACON AND TOMATO SWEET POTATO

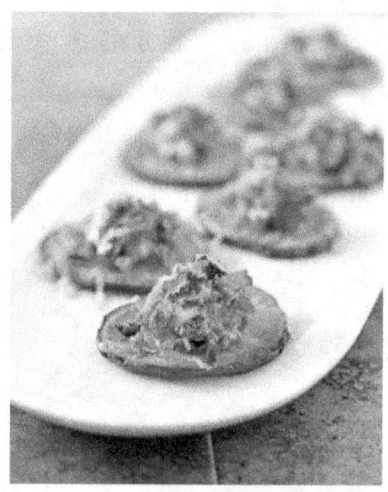

**Ingredients:**

Two sweet potato

Two tbsp. of olive oil

Two cups of cherry or grape or tomatoes can fit as well. It is necessary to cut into quarters.

Six slices of a bacon, it is necessary to cook it and make crispy

A bit of a freshly chopped parsley

A bit of a sea salt on your taste

A bit of a black pepper on your taste

# Paleo Diet for Beginners:

80 Healthy Paleo Recipes and 31 Proven Steps to Loose Weight

**Instructions:**

1. Put a special pepper on a baking sheet, also preheat the broiler. Cut the sweet potatoes and put it onto the baking sheet.

2. Sprinkle with olive oil and salt. Broil until it is cooked.

3. Mix together the tomatoes and the cooked bacon add parsley. Add fresh ground pepper and also put the slices onto the sweet potato before serving.

## 45. BLUEBERRY COCONUT CEREALS

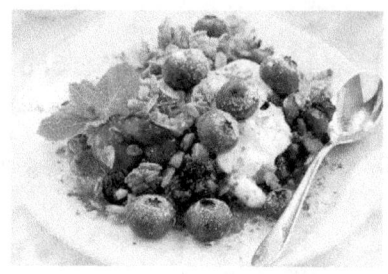

**Ingredients:**

two cups of chopped pecans

one third cup of coconut oil

six or seven dates

one cup of pumpkin seeds

one tbsp. of vanilla

two tbsp. of cinnamon

a half of tsp of sea salt

one half of coconut flakes, unsweetened

one half of blueberries

**Instructions:**
1.  Heat the oven to 325F.
2.  Put pecans, coconut oil, dates in a food processor. Mix everything up thoroughly
3.  Add the pecans and pumpkin seeds and ground everything thoroughly as well.
4.  Put to a bowl and put some vanilla, cinnamon and salt. Stir and spread on a baking sheet.

5. Bake for approximately twenty minutes, until browned. Take away, let them cool, and stir in the coconut and blueberries.

## 46. CHOCOLATE COCONUT DROPS

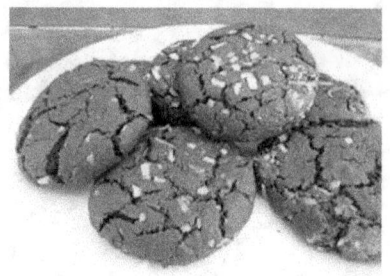

### Ingredients:

three tbsp of coconut oil

one and a half of dark chocolate chips

one and a half of cocoa powder

two tbsp. of honey

less than a half of almond butter

one cup of coconut flakes

### Instructions:

1. Put the chocolate chips and coconut oil in the microwave. Cook in thirty minutes intervals until you see that the chips are melted.
2. Put the coconut oil and chocolate chips in a microwave safe bowl. Cook in 30 second intervals until chips are melted, stirring between each interval.
3. Stir all the cocoa powder plus honey, and almond butter. When everything is smooth, add the coconut and stir until well perfectly.
4. Put a baking sheet with special. Put into the fridge until cookies are steady.

## 47. MINI FLOURLESS CHOCOLATE CAKES

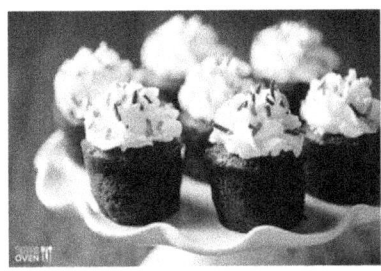

### Ingredients:

Two bananas;

One egg;

Two table spoon of honey;

four table spoon of dark cocoa powder;

vannila on the edge of a spoon

two table spoons of sliced almonds;

### Instructions:

Heat the oven to 375 F.
Stir together all ingredients using the blender
Pour the liquid into two separate bowls; put almonds on the top.
Bake for twenty - five minutes approximately.

## 48. PUMPKIN COOKIES

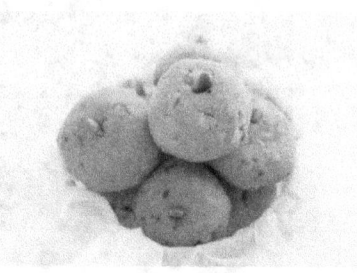

**Ingredients:**

One cup of pumpkin puree;

Less than a half of a cup applesauce;

Less than a half of coconut milk

One teaspoon of vanilla

one cup of almond meal;

a half of a cup of coconut flour;

a half of a tea spoon of pumpkin pie spice;


**Instructions:**

Heat the oven to 350 F.
Put the applesauce, coconut milk, pumpkin puree, coconut milk in a bowl. Mix everything well.
Then add the coconut flour and almond meal and stir everything well as well.
On a baking sheet put the parchment and put the batter on it with the help of a spoon.
Place the baking sheet in the oven and leave it there for thirty minutes or so.

## 49. PALEO GRANOLA

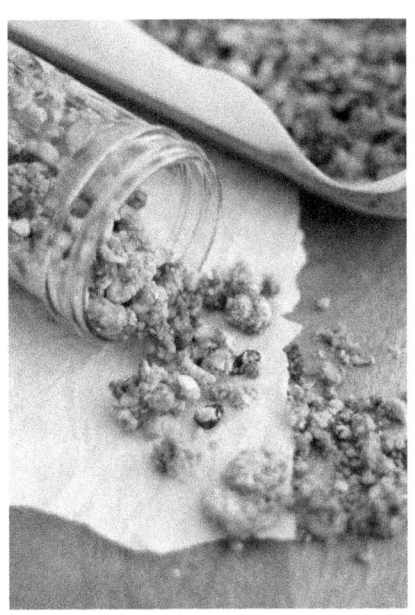

**Ingredients:**

Raw almonds - 140 g

Raw cashews - 140 g

Raw pumpkin seeds (shelled) - 35 g

Raw sunflower seeds (shelled) - 35 g

Unsweetened coconut flakes - 70 g

Coconut oil - 60 ml

Honey - 120 ml

# Paleo Diet for Beginners:

80 Healthy Paleo Recipes and 31 Proven Steps to Loose Weight

Powdered vanillin - one tsp.

Sea salt - one tsp.

Raisins (or any dried fruits) - 140 g

**Instructions:**

1. Heat  the oven to 135 C in advance.
2. Grind seeds, almonds, cashews  in a blender for several minutes.
3. Mix soft butter, coconut oil, honey and powered vanilla in a medium sized saucepan. Let all components melt over medium-high heat.
4. Add the ground nut mixture and stir well.
5. Take a baking sheet,  line it  with pergament paper and pour the granola mixture.
6  Do brown during 20-25 minutes.
 7. Take finished granola  out of the oven. Spread the raisins or dried fruits and sea salt .
8.  Press the mixture together. Form a flat,  tight surface.
9.  Cool for about 20-30 minutes. Cut into and chunks.
10. You may store granola  in an sealed container for about a week.

## 50. PALEO NUT ENERGY BARS

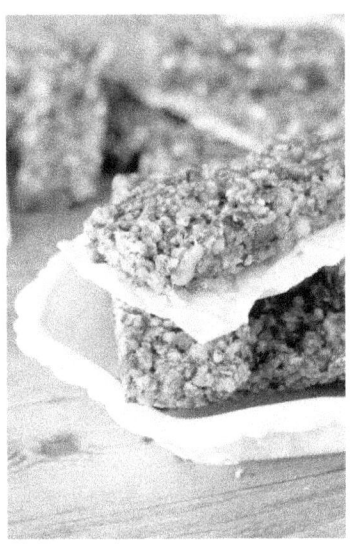

**Ingredients:**

Chopped pecans - 200 g

Chopped walnuts - 100 g

Chopped almonds - 100 g

Dates - 20 pcs

Liquid egg whites - 250 g

Cinnamon - two tblsp.

Powdered vanillin - 1,5 tsp

**Instructions:**

1. Preheat the oven to 175 C.
2. Take a large cup and combine all components.

3.  Prepare the dish for baking.  Line it with pergament paper or aluminum leaf and oil it. Pour out the nut mixture on a dish and press well.

4. Bake for about fifteen-sixteen minutes.

5. Remove energy nut bars from the oven.

6. Let them to get cool for five  minutes.

6.  Slice the bars.

7. Enjoy bars and energize for the whole day!

## 51. Homemade Strawberry Fruit Leather

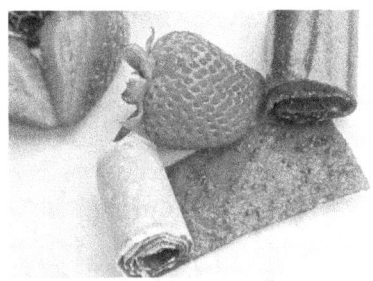

**Ingredients:**

Chopped strawberries – 400 g

Honey - two tbsp.

**Instructions:**

1. Heat the oven to 80 C.
2. Put a silpat mat on the baking sheet.  Spread berries in a pan and bake at 80 C until soft. Fold in two tablespoons of  honey and stir well.
3.  Puree the strawberries   until smooth.
4. Pour honey-strawberries mixture onto the silpat baking mat.
5. Do not raise the temperature  and bake for 6-7 hours.
6. When strawberry  leather is ready, it should peel away from the silpat mat.
7. Take a knife or scissors to cut this yummy  leather into strips.
8. Make rolls to serve!
9. You may store fruit leather in a hermetically sealed package or container.

**Paleo Breakfast recipes**

## 52. WEEKEND WARRIOR OMELETTE

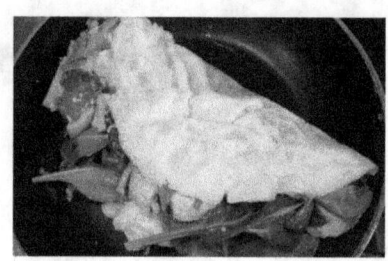

### Ingredients:

Organic eggs – 2 pcs

Olive oil - 1 tsp

Green onions – 2 pcs

Organic spinach leaves – 6 pcs

Organic tomatoes – 2 pcs

Half an organic avocado

### Instructions:

1. Heat olive oil in a shallow pan.
2.  Dice onions and sauté it for 5 minutes.
3. Scramble eggs and pour to onion.
4. Fry for about two minutes.
4. Add diced avocado, tomatoes and salt to taste.
5. Fold in half and turn over  melette until it  fully cooked.
6. Put the scrambled eggs on spinach leaves
7.  Enjoy!

## 53. ROSEMARY ORANGE DUCK WITH ROASTED VEGETABLES

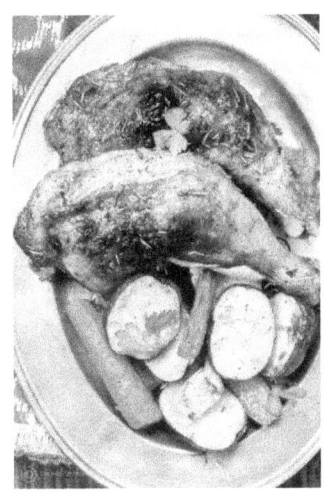

**Ingredients:**

One big duck

Oranges – two- three pcs

Bunch of rosemary – 1 piece

Carrot – 5-6 pcs

Pasternak – 5-6 pcs

Leek – 3 pcs

Garlic bulblet - 3 pcs

Ground black pepper

**Instructions:**

# Paleo Diet for Beginners:

80 Healthy Paleo Recipes and 31 Proven Steps to Loose Weight

1. Take three garlic bulblets, peel and crush them.  Wash, peel and chop the carrots and pasternak. Cut three leeks into small rounds.

2. Mix chopped vegetables and add crushed garlic. Thereafter spread this savory blend on the greased bottom of a firepan

3. Take a dressed duck. Wash it and dry with a paper towel. Salt and pepper. If you like, you can slightly spread crushed garlic on the carcass of the duck .

4. Cut two or three oranges into four pieces. Stuff a duck with oranges and rosemary.

5. Put  the carcass of the duck on top of the vegetables.

6. Heat the oven to 190 C and place the firepan in it.  The duck bakes about three hours. BUT Every 20 minutes take your duck with vegetables out of the oven to water the juice over it. This helps keep it from drying out.

Three hours later, your rosemary orange duck with roasted vegetables will be ready!
It smells delicious!  Taste it!

## 54. MEMORIAL DAY PALEO GRILLING MARINADES

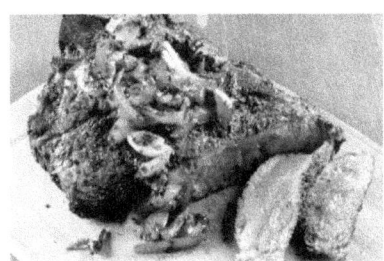

**Ingredients:**

Melted coconut oil – 1cup

Freshly squeezed Meyer lemon juice – two tbsp

Honey – 1,5 tbsp

A small piece of fresh ginger root

Paprika

Fresh ground black pepper – 0,5 tsp

A pinch of crushed red chili flakes

Garlic bulblet - 5 pcs

Finely chopped spring onion – 3 pcs

**Instructions:**

1. Take a food processor bowl and put there all ingredients for marinade (except spring onion)
2. Mix thoroughly to reach a homogeneous consistency
3. Spread the marinade on the fish fillet and put into the bowl.
4 The fish is marinated for 30 minutes.
5. Then take it out of the bowl and cook in grill basket.

6. Sprinkle grilled fish with spring onion. Enjoy!

## 55. SAVORY MEAT

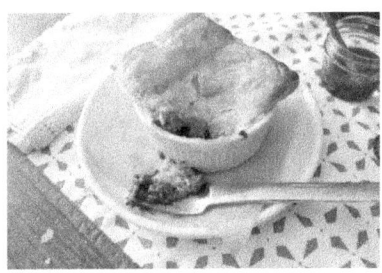

**Ingredients:**

Freshly squeezed lime juice – 50 ml

Duck fat – three tbsp

Freshly squeezed lemon juice – 15 ml

Ground black pepper

Cumin – one tsp

Garlic bulblet - 4 pcs

Hungarian paprika – one tbsp

Shallot – 2 pcs

Thyme – one tsp.

**Instructions:**

1. Take a food processor bowl and put there all ingredients. Mix thoroughly to reach a homogeneous consistency.
2. Choose any grass fed meat you like (beet, chicken, goat, turkey etc)
3. Marinade the meat.
4. The meat is marinated for one day
5. Prepare any way you like!

## 56. SWEET SAVORY MEAT

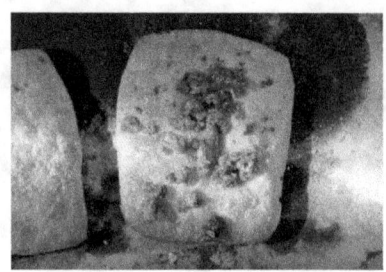

**Ingredients:**

Orange – 1 piece

Orange zest – one tsp

Melted coconut oil – one cup

Oregano – one tbsp

Freshly squeezed lime juice – 2-3 tbsp

Jalapeno – one piece, seeds removed*

Garlic bulbet – two pcs

Fresh cilantro leaves - 1/2 cup

**Instructions:**

1. Take a food processor bowl and put there all ingredients. Mix thoroughly to reach a homogeneous consistency.
2. Choose any grass fed meat you like (beet, chicken, goat, turkey etc)
3.  Spread the marinade on the meat and put into the bowl.
4. The meat is marinated for one day
5. Prepare  any way you like!

## PALEO DINNER RECIPES

# 57. PIZZA SOUP

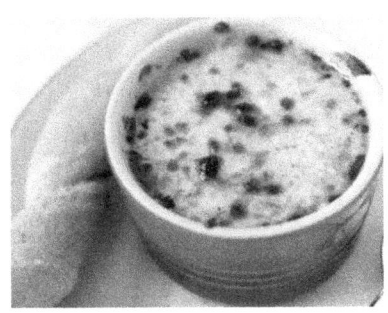

## Ingredients:

Sliced chicken sausage – 340 g

Marinara – one jar (700g)

Pepperoni – 115 g (cut into four pieces)

Fire roasted tomatoes – one can (400 g)

Onion – one piece

Sliced mushrooms – 450 g

Sliced black olives – one can (370 g)

Dried oregano – one tbsp

Powdered garlic – one tsp

Salt – 0,5 tsp

## Instructions:

# Paleo Diet for Beginners:

80 Healthy Paleo Recipes and 31 Proven Steps to Loose Weight

1. Take a deep, large saucepan. Put sliced chicken sausage, pepperoni, marinara, one can of fire roasted tomatoes, onion, sliced mushrooms, black olives, one tablespoon of dried oregano, one teaspoon of powdered garlic and salt.
2. Boil over low heat for 30 minutes. Mushrooms and onion should be soft.
3. Add salt if necessary.
4. Your pizza soup is ready!
5. Serve hot!

## 58. Easy Sweet and Sour Pork

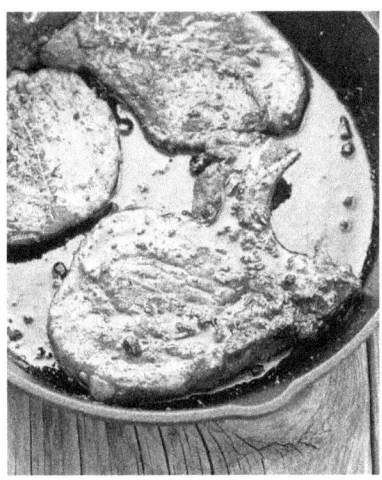

**Ingredients:**

Bone-in pork chops (225 g each) – four pcs

Butte – two tbspr

Ground black pepper

Salt – one tsp

Balsamic vinegar – two tbsp

Honey - two tbsp

Chopped garlic bulbet – two pcs

Dried rosemary – 0,5 tsp

Dried oregano – 0,5 tsp

Red pepper flakes

# Paleo Diet for Beginners:

80 Healthy Paleo Recipes and 31 Proven Steps to Loose Weight

## Instructions:

1. Heat oven to 200°C.
2. Salt and pepper pork chops. Let marinade.
3. Take the required amount of butter. Melt it on a slow fire.
4. Place pork chops and fry on both sides until browned (2 min per side).
5. Transfer the pan in the oven.
6. Roast for about six minutes.

GLAZE

1. Take a bowl and mix components for glaze.
2. Transfer this spicy mixture into the saucepan. Let it cook slowly (about 5 min).

Back to the chops

1. Remove browned roasted chops from the oven, pour spicy glaze over the top. Back in the oven.
2. Bake for four-five min until caramelized.
3. Serve hot!

## 59. Spicy Tuna and Tomato Burgers

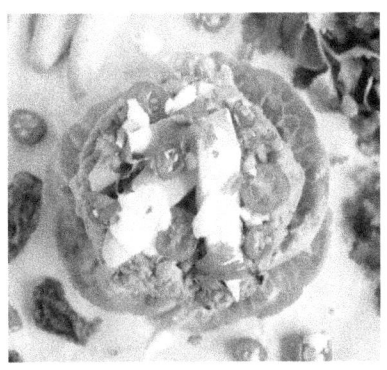

**Ingredients:**

Tuna – (1x 95g can)

Red onion – one piece

Red chilli – one small piece

Garlic bulbet – one piece

Egg  - one piece

Tomato paste – two tbsps

Coconut flour – one tbsp

Salt and pepper

Fresh coriander

Lettuce leaves

Avocado

Sour cream (or Greek yoghurt )

# Paleo Diet for Beginners:

80 Healthy Paleo Recipes and 31 Proven Steps to Loose Weight

## Instructions:

1. Heat the oven to 175'C
2. Use wax paper to line a baking tray.
3. Drain and rinse tuna, chop red onion and red chili, crush garlic bulbets.
4 .Toss to combine all ingredients for burger in a bowl .
5.  Divide tuna mass into six small sized burgers and put onto prepared baking tray.
6. Place the tray in the oven. Bake for 10 mins, until ready..
7 .Serve with fresh juicy lettuce leaves , sliced avocado, add one tbsp of   sour cream  (or greek yoghurt ) and drizzle with some fresh coriander, salt, pepper  and slices of red chilli.
8. Enjoy!

## 60. Tomato Basil Cauliflower Rice

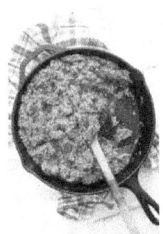

**Ingredients:**

Cauliflower – one head

Dried Oregano one tsp

Dried Basil – 1,5 tsp

Marjoram – 0,5 tsp

Powdered onion – 0,5 tsp

Chopped garlic – 0,5 tsp

Black pepper

Unsalted tomato paste – 85 g

Dried parsley

**Instructions:**

1. Divide cauliflower into small curds. Grind in a food processor
2. Take a deep stewing pan and put there the cauliflower and the rest of the components. Stew gently for a further 5-8 mins
3. Remove and serve!

## 61. Chicken with Cauliflower and Olives

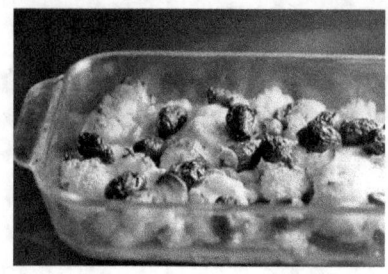

**Ingredients:**

Chicken breast – 450 g (boneless, skinless)

Thyme sprigs – 1 bunch

Cauliflower – one head (divide into curds)

Shallot – 1 piece

Olive oil - 3 tblsp

Sea salt

Black pepper

Zest of one lemon

Fresh lemon juice - ¼ cup

Kalamata olives - 1 cup, pitted

Garlic bulbet – 5 pcs,

**Instructions:**

1. Wash chicken breast and dry itl.
2. Take some thyme sprigs and place in the baking dish
3. Put chicken breast and cauliflower curds over the thyme sprigs.

4. Take a deep bowl to mix finely chopped shallot, pepper, salt, lemon zest, olive oil, juice, pitted olives and thinly sliced garlic

5. Marinate chicken and cauliflower curds in lemon mixture for a day..

6. Bake chicken with cauliflower curds and olives at 200° for one hour until well browned

7. Serve hot!

## 62. Sesame Salmon Burgers

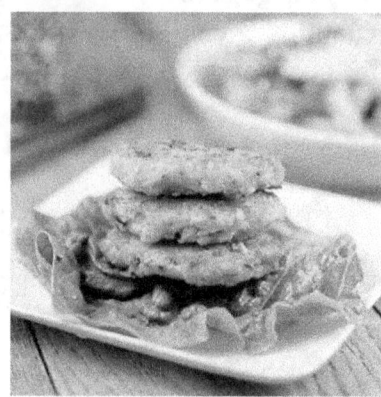

**Ingredients:**

Salmon -  450 g (skinned)

Egg – 2 pcs

Toasted sesame seeds – 50 g

Toasted sesame oil – 20 ml

Ume plum vinegar – 15 ml

Garlic bulbet - 1 piece ( pressed)

Fresh ginger – 5 g (peeled and minced)

Spring onion

Coconut flour – 20 g

Coconut oil

# Paleo Diet for Beginners:

80 Healthy Paleo Recipes and 31 Proven Steps to Loose Weight

**Instructions:**

1. Rinse the fish, pat dry and cut into cubes
2. Take a large bowl. Mix toasted sesame oil, ume plum vinegar, pressed garlic, minced ginger, chopped spring onion, toasted sesame seeds and two eggs. Place pieces of salmon in this marinade. Add coconut flour. Stir all ingredients thoroughly.
3. Form small patties.
4. Take a skillet, pour coconut oil in it and heat.
5. Fry the patties until golden brown
6. Put the patties on a paper towel.
7. Serve hot with vegetable puree!

## 63. Green Chili Turkey Burgers

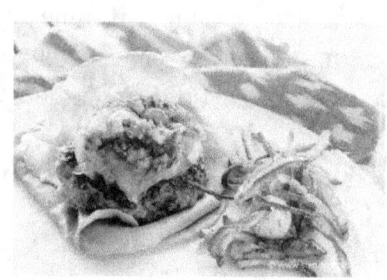

**Ingredients:**

Diced green chilies (2 cansx112 g)

Ground turkey meat – 450 g

Cilantro – 50 g

Onion – 30 g

Chili powder – 5 g

Cumin – 10 g

Sea salt

**Instructions:**

1. Prepare a dry big bowl. Put there ground turkey meat and mix with diced green chilies,finely chopped cilantro, onion add salt, chili powder and cumin.
2. Form 8 medium-sized patties and grill them.
3. Serve hot with vegetable puree!

## 64. Roasted Chicken With Olives And Prunes

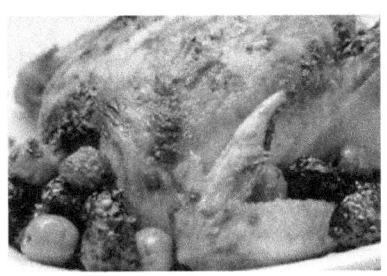

**Ingredients:**

Dressed chicken – 900-1300 g

Green olives - 150 g (pitted)

Prunes – 150 g (pitted)

Capers – 20 g

Dried oregano – 20 g

Honey – 85 g

Bay leaves – two pcs

Garlic bulbet - 1 piece

Olive oil – 60 ml

Apple vinegar – 60 ml

Water – 60 ml

Sea salt

# Paleo Diet for Beginners:

80 Healthy Paleo Recipes and 31 Proven Steps to Loose Weight

**Instructions:**

1. Wash the chicken and pat dry with paper towel.
2. Put the chicken in the baking tray then drizzle with salt
3. Take a large bowl and mix the pitted olives and prunes, 20 g of oregano, 20 g of capers, two flavorous bay leaves, pressed garlic, 60 ml of olive oil and apple vinegar, 60 ml of water. Stir thoroughly.
4. Pour this spicy mixture in the tray around the chicken.
5. Roast the chicken at 220°C for twenty minutes
6. Reduce temperature to 180°C and continue to bake the chicken until until golden crisp (about forty minutes)
7. Take a flavorous, juicy chicken out of the oven and serve.

## 65. Shrimp Cakes

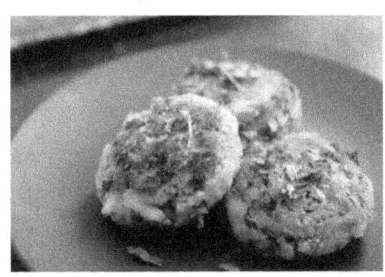

**Ingredients:**

Raw shrimps – 450 g

Egg – one piece

Blanched almond flour – 60 g

Red or yellow bell pepper – one piece

Garlic bulbet – 1 piece

Green onion – two tbsp

Grapeseed oil – 15 ml

Lime juice – 15 ml

Agave nectar – 15 ml

Cilantro – 40 g

Chipotle chile – 2 g

Sea salt

# Paleo Diet for Beginners:

80 Healthy Paleo Recipes and 31 Proven Steps to Loose Weight

**Instructions:**

1. Chop raw peeled shrimps in kitchen machine.
2. Take a large bowl and mix chopped shrimps, finely chopped bell pepper, minced garlic, thinly sliced green onion, 15 ml of lime juice, 15 ml of agave nectar, salt, 2 g of chipotle chile, one egg and 40 g of finely chopped cilantro
3. Form 12 thick patties of this mixture and roll in almond flour.
4. Take a large non-stick frying pan, pour 15 ml of oil and heat it.
5. Fry patties on both sides until golden brown (about 5 minutes per side).
6. Line a paper towel on the dish and put the patties on it.
7. Serve with vegetable puree!

## 66. Curried Prawns

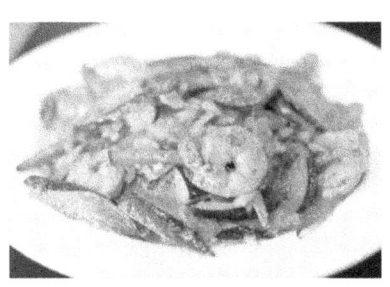

**Ingredients:**

Large prawns – 450 g

Tomato puree – 120 g

Olive oil – 60 ml

Garlic bulbet – 4 pcs

Onion – 1 piece

Ginger - 40 g

Cumin - ½ tsp

Coriander - ½ tsp

Turmeric -½ tsp

Cilantro -1 bunch

Fresh lime juice – 45 ml

# Paleo Diet for Beginners:

80 Healthy Paleo Recipes and 31 Proven Steps to Loose Weight

**Instructions:**
1. Pour olive oil in an enamel pot and heat it.
2. Take peeled and chopped garlic, onion and sauté until tender. Add tomato puree and spices ginger; stew for 5 minutes
3. Put the prawns in the boiling sauce and cook up to readiness (10 minutes).
4. Add finely chopped cilantro. Mix thoroughly.
5. Place on the dish and drizzle with lime juice
6. It is incredibly delicious!

## 67. Lebanese Lemon Chicken

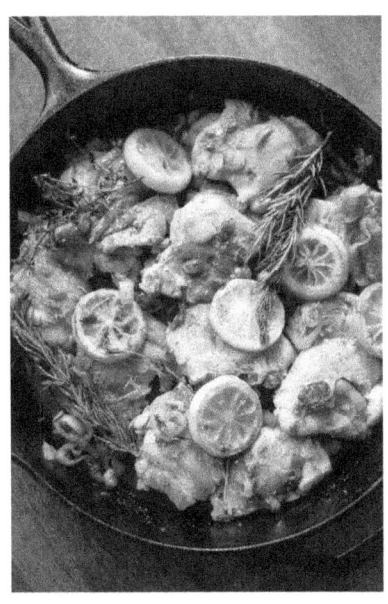

**Ingredients:**

Chicken thighs – 12 pcs (boneless, skinless)

Olive oil – three tbsp

Organic lemons – three pcs

Lemon – 3 pcs

Curcuma – 0, 5 tsp

Onion – 1 piece

Sea salt – 1, 5 tsp

Ground black pepper

Sprigs of rosemary – 2 pcs

Sprigs of thyme – 2 pcs

**Instructions:**
1. Take two tbsps of lemon juice. Pour juice in a large bowl, add two tablespoons of olive oil, 0,5 teaspoon of curcuma, sea salt and black pepper.
2. Marinade chicken thighs.
3. Slice two lemons and onion.
4. Take a large cast iron skillet, pour an olive oil and heat it
5. Put chicken thighs and fry on both sides for 8 minutes
6. Transfer fried thighs to a plate.
7. Put lemon and onion slices, herbs in the pan. Let stew for several minutes
8. Then pour 50 g of water into the pan and put the chicken back.
9. Stew chicken with mixture of lemon, herbs and onion for 10 minutes.
10. Flavorful lebanese lemon chicken is ready!
11. Better serve with rice or cauliflower rice.

## 68. Paleo Chicken Bowl

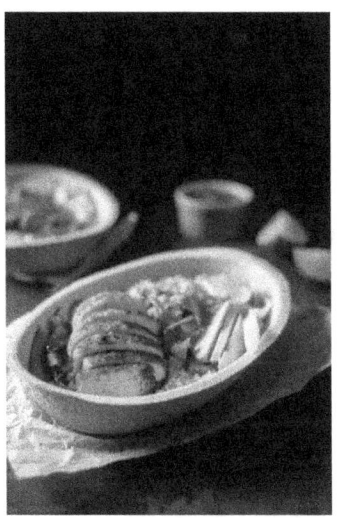

**Ingredients:**

Avocado – 2 pcs

Roasted peppers - 1 jar (335 g)

Garlic bulbet - 2 pcs

Chicken thighs – 500 g (boneless, skinless)

Olive oil – 15ml

Red onion - one small

Sliced mushrooms – 300 g

Greens (any you like)

Salt and pepper

# Paleo Diet for Beginners:

80 Healthy Paleo Recipes and 31 Proven Steps to Loose Weight

**Instructions:**
Make roasted pepper sauce
1. Take one avocado, drained roasted peppers, mashed garlic, salt and pepper. Put all ingredients into a kitchen machine. Mix until smooth and let the sauce cool.
Cook chicken
1. Do up chicken with salt and pepper. Take a large skillet, heat it and add olive oil. Fry chicken thighs brown on both sides..
2. While frying, peel and dice vegetables and greens.
3. Transfer the finished chicken to the dish.
4. Fry onion about 1-2 minutes, then add mushrooms and fry 2-3 minutes. Add greens and fry again about 1-2 minutes.
5. Divide the chicken into small portions and mix with fried vegetables.
6. Put into bowls.
8. Serve with roasted pepper sauce.

## 69. Paleo Baked Eggs in Tomatoes

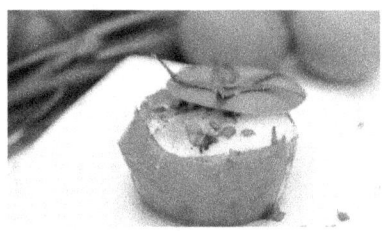

**Ingredients:**

Tomatoes in own juice – 1200 ml

Powdered garlic

Black pepper bacon – 6 slices

Organic eggs – 12 pcs

Chopped green onions – 3 pcs

Sea salt

**Instructions:**
1. Heat the oven to 180°C.
2. Pour tomatoes in own juice in a glass dish).
3. Mash the tomatoes. Season with powdered garlic and mix with the sliced black pepper bacon. Stir spicy tomato sauce thoroughly.
4. Break the eggs into this sauce (not scramble).
5. Drizzle with green and give relish to a dish (use pepper and salt.
6. Put it in the oven. Cook for 60 minutes.
7. Take ready baked eggs in tomatoes out of the oven.
8. Enjoy!

## 70. Indian Spiced Brussels & Carrots

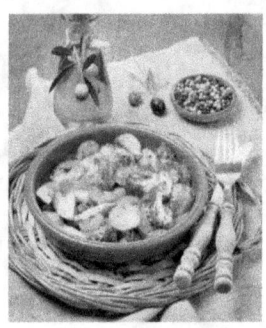

**Ingredients:**

Brussels sprouts – 1 kg
Carrots – 2 pcs , peeled & sliced
Garam masala
Sweet curry
Coriander
Coarse ground sea salt
Avocado oil

**Instructions:**
1. Prepare the oven. Heat it to 200°C.
2. Prepare the brussels sprouts: chop the ends off, cut damaged outer peel
3. Cut the sprouts into equal parts. Spread these pieces into casserole dish
4. Add peeled and  sliced carrot and season  to taste. Sprinkle with avocado oil and mix thoroughly.
5. Put the dish to the oven and cook for 20 minutes.
6. Mix again and bake for 20-30 minutes  until do brown.
7. Take the dish out of the oven.
8. Enjoy warm!

# Paleo Diet for Beginners:

80 Healthy Paleo Recipes and 31 Proven Steps to Loose Weight

**Paleo Smoothie Recipes**

# 71. Very Berry Smoothie

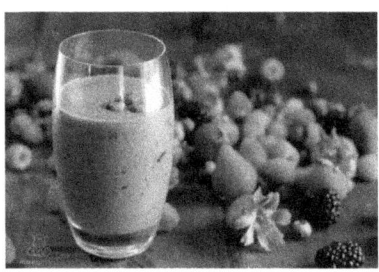

**Ingredients:**

Spinach - 2 cups

Mixed berries - 200-220 g

Frozen bananas – 1 piece

Peeled kiwi - 1 piece

Water - 480 ml

**Instructions:**
1. Blend spinach, berries, bananas, kiwi and water until smooth.
2. Enjoy your very berry smoothie.

## 72. Strawberry Banana Smoothie

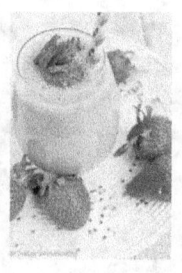

**Ingredients:**

Diced fresh strawberries – 100-170 g

Banana – 1 piece

Almond milk - 120 ml

Cube ice -200 g

Honey - 1/2 tbsp

**Instructions:**
1. Mix all of the components. Make a purée in blender until smooth.
2. If your smoothie is so thick – pour some almond milk to get your favorite consistency.
3. Put 0, 5 tbsp of honey (or more if necessary).
4. Drink immediately.

## 73. Mango Lime Smoothie

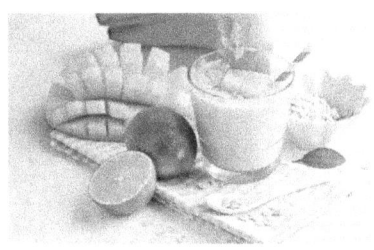

**Ingredients:**

Freshly squeezed lime juice - two tbsp

Spinach - 2 cups

Frozen mango – 250 g

**Instructions:**
1. Mix all of the components. Make a purée in blender until smooth
2. Help yourself!

## 74. Cinnamon Chia Smoothie

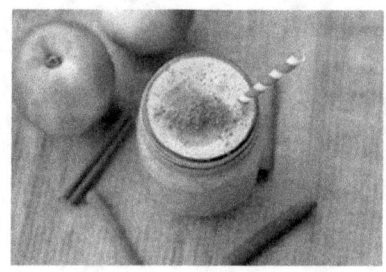

### Ingredients:

Almond milk - 240 ml

Spinach - 1 cup

Peeled apple – 1 piece

Chia seeds – two tbsps

Maple syrup – one tbsp

Cinnamon - 0, 5 tbsp

### Instructions:
1. Mix thoroughly all ingredients. Whisk until smooth.
2. Sprinkle smoothie with chia seeds
3. Enjoy this cinnamon chia smoothie!

## 75. Almond Cantaloupe Smoothie

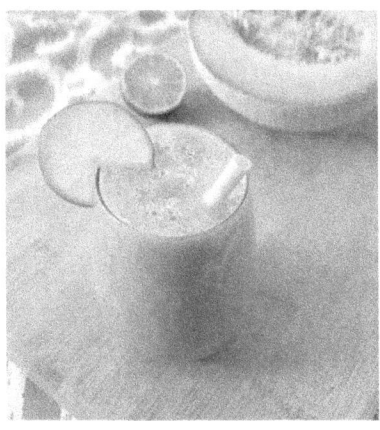

**Ingredients:**

Spinach – 250 g

Unsweetened almond milk – 240 ml

Mixed berries - 200-220 g

Sweet and peeled cantaloupe -   1/2

Water – 120 ml

Cube ice

**Instructions:**
1. Whisk all ingredients until smooth.
2. Pour in a glass with fresh smoothie several ice cubes.
3. Enjoy this tasty and healthy cool drink!

## 76. Paleo Desserts cookies recipes

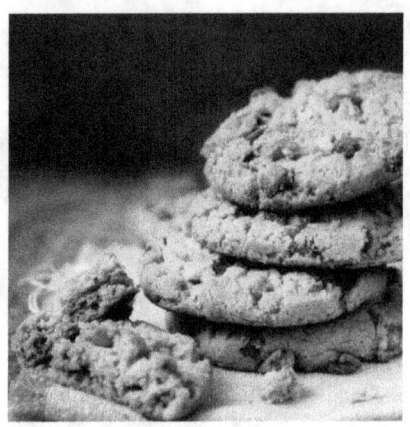

**Ingredients:**

 Almond butter - 225 g

Almonds- 100 g

Rich coconut milk – 240 ml

Unsweetened shredded coconut – 200 g

Fresh eggs – 3 pieces

A pinch of powered vanillin

Honey – two tbsp

Gel- molding frames - 1 package

**Instructions:**
1. Preheat oven to 400 F.
2. Combine all components.
3. Pour into gel- molding frames for muffins
4. Bake about 15 minutes.

## 77. Nut free banana bread

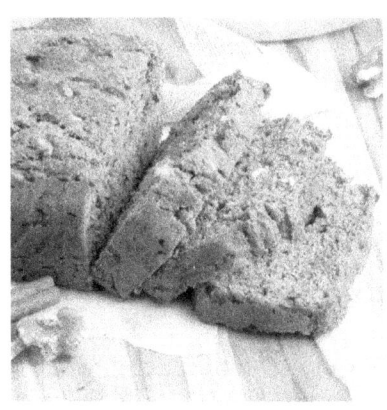

**Ingredients:**

Puree of one banana

Fresh eggs – 2 pcs

Sunflower seed butter peanut butter – 170 g

Maple syrup – 120 ml

Powered vanillin – one tbsp

Fresh lemon juice – 15 ml

Coconut oil – 30 ml

Starch (tapioca flour) - 70 g

Cinnamon - one tsp

Ground ginger (to taste)

Baking powder – one tsp

Tartar sauce – 5 ml

Ground nutmeg (to taste)

Sea salt

**Instructions:**

1. Preheat oven to 180 C.
2. Grease a loaf pan with 1 tbsp of coconut oil. Take a piece of wax paper and put it on the bottom of baking form. Grease wax paper with coconut oil too.
3. Take a bowl, mix together the tapioca flour, nutmeg, baking soda and add cinnamon, ginger, Tartar sauce and salt. Stir well.
4. Take a blender and mix puree of one banana, two eggs, 120 ml of maple syrup, 170 g of sunflower seeds butter, powered vanillin, lemon juice and coconut oil. Whisk carefully.
5. Add mixture of dry ingredients to the blender and beat until batter.
6. Remove the batter from the bowl and pour into the baking form.
7. Bake for 55-60 minutes until golden crust.
8. Let the dish to cool.
9. Slice as you like and enjoy!

## 78. Carrot Banana Muffins (for 12 servings)

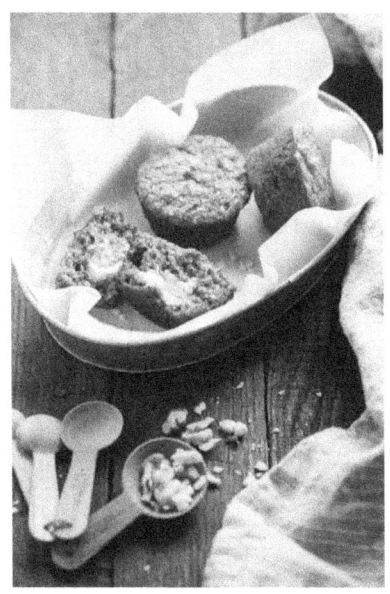

**Ingredients:**

Almond flour – 280 g

Baking powder – two tsp

Cinnamon - one tsp

Pitted dates – 100 g

Bananas – 3 pcs

Fresh eggs – 3 pcs

Cider vinegar – one tsp

Shredded carrot – 150 g

# Paleo Diet for Beginners:

80 Healthy Paleo Recipes and 31 Proven Steps to Loose Weight

Finely chopped nuts (any kind of nut you like)

Gel- molding frames - 1 package

Melted coconut oil – 57 g

Sea salt

**Instructions:**

1. Heat oven to 180 C.
2. Take a deep, dry bowl to mix ingredients in accordance with the recipe (flour, a pinch of salt, baking powder and one teaspoon of cinnamon.
3. Combine bananas, eggs, dates, coconut oil, cider vinegar in a kitchen machine.
4. Join mixture from kitchen machine to dry components in the deep bowl. Whisk it thoroughly.
5. Add 150 g of shredded carrot and finely chopped nuts.
6. Move the batter from the bowl and pour into gel-molding frames for muffins.
7. Bake for 25 minute at 180 C
8. Here are your muffins - enjoy!

## 79. Fresh Zucchini Bread

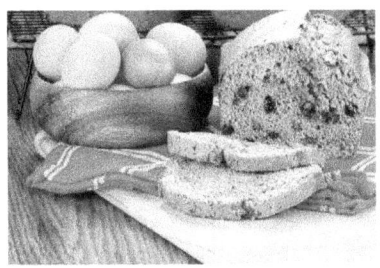

**Ingredients:** (per 8 servings)

One large grated zucchini

Kosher salt – 0, 5 tsp

Almond flour – 210 g

Baking powder – one tsp

Cinnamon - two tsps

Ground nutmeg (to taste)

Fresh eggs – 2 pcs

Melted coconut oil – 60 ml

Powered vanillin – one tbsp

Raw honey - 85 g

**Instructions:**
1. Heat oven to 180 C.
2. Grate one large zucchini. Add to this mass some salt and let sit for five minutes.
3. Pour away the excess water.
4. Combine dry components together. Mix well.

5. Take another bowl and blend eggs, powered vanillin, the coconut oil and honey. Spread this mixture into the dry components. Blend and add to zucchini.

6. Grease a cake tin with coconut oil, and pour the batter into it.

7. Bake about 35-45 minutes until do brown.

8. Let the zucchini bread to cool.

9. Slice it and enjoy!

## 80. Paleo Carrot Cake

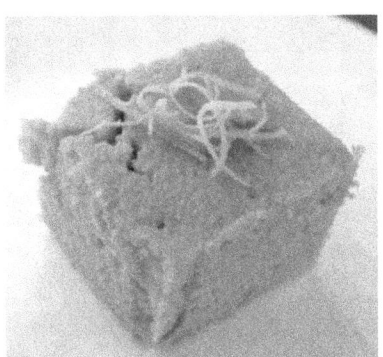

**Ingredients:**

Almond flour – 210 g

Coconut flour – 46 g

Arrowroot powder – 140 g

Cinnamon - one tbls

Baking powder – two tsp

Baking soda – one tsp

Maple syrup or honey – 170 g

Melted coconut oil – 3/4   cup

Powered vanillin – one tbsp

Orange zest – one tbsp

Grated carrot – three pcs(s)

Sea salt (to taste)

Ground ginger (to taste)

Ground nutmeg (to taste)

Eggs – 9 pcs

**Glaze Ingredients:**

Soaked cashews – 1 cup

Coconut oil - 13/4 cup

Coconut butter – 113 g

Fresh lemon juice – one tbsp

Maple syrup – 85 g

Powered vanillin – one tbsp vanilla

Cider vinegar – two tbsp

**Instructions:**
*Bake the cake.*

1. Heat oven to 180 C.  Grease baking case with coconut oil.

2. Mix dry ingredients.

3. Take another bowl, mix wet ingredients (except carrots) and blend.

4. Empty   dry mixture out of the dish and add to the wet. Stir well.

5. Put grated carrot. Pour the batter into prepared baking case.

6. Bake for 30-35 minutes until do brown.

7. Let the cake to cool down.

*Make the glaze*

1. Drain the cashews. Blend until creamy.

2. Put the rest ingredients for glaze and beat until creamy

# Paleo Diet for Beginners:

80 Healthy Paleo Recipes and 31 Proven Steps to Loose Weight

3. Put the glaze over the cake.

4. Carrot cake is ready! Cut it and serve!

# Paleo Diet for Beginners:

## 80 Healthy Paleo Recipes and 31 Proven Steps to Loose Weight

Thank You!

I am very happy that you have chosen this book and it's been a real pleasure writing it for you. My aim is to help as many readers as possible. So many of us are able to take new knowledge and use it to our lives with really useful and long lasting consequences and it is my desire that you have been able to take value from the information I have written.

Thank you for beeing with me during this book and for reading it through to the end. I really hope that you have enjoyed the information and that's why I appreciate your thoughts on my material so much. If you could take a couple of minutes to write a feedback, your views will help me to create more material that you find beneficial.

Thanks again for your attention. I really look forward to reading your review.

Stay Healthy!

# Paleo Diet for Beginners:

80 Healthy Paleo Recipes and 31 Proven Steps to Loose Weight

## BY THE SAME AUTHOR

**You are welcome to read another useful and very informative book by this author!**

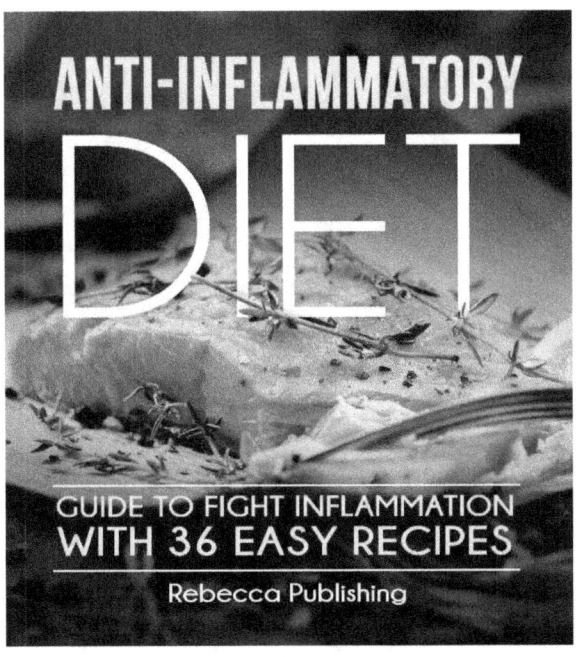

**Please search this page over the www.amazon.com**

www.amazon.com/s/ref=nb_sb_noss?url=search-alias%3Daps&field-keywords=B0718WKD81